2024 GLYCEMIC INDEX & LOAD DIET FOR DIABETES

EASY SCIENCE-BASED MEAL PLANS WITH GI, GL & CARB COUNTER, AND EXTENSIVE DIABETES-FRIENDLY FOOD LISTS

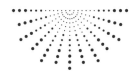

DR. H. MAHER

Medical Disclaimer:

Accuracy and Diligence:

The author and publisher of "2024 Glycemic Index & Load Diet for Diabetes " have made every effort to ensure the accuracy and completeness of the information provided within this publication. Extensive research and careful consideration have been employed to present data and insights that reflect the latest and most relevant information available up to the date of publication.

Use of Up-to-Date Information:

This book incorporates the latest data and insights available in the field of nutrition and diabetes management at the time of writing. The author and publisher are committed to using the most current and scientifically validated information to support the recommendations and advice provided herein.

General Information:

The dieting and nutritional guidance offered in this book is intended for informational purposes only and does not constitute medical advice, diagnosis, treatment, or any other professional healthcare advice. Due to the unique nature of each individual's health conditions and nutritional needs, the content may not be appropriate for everyone.

Consultation with Healthcare Professionals:

It is crucial for readers to consult with their physician or another qualified healthcare professional before initiating any new dieting, weight loss, or exercise program, especially those with pre-existing health conditions, those under medical treatment, or individuals with specific dietary needs and restrictions. Continuous supervision by a healthcare provider is recommended to ensure the safety and appropriateness of any dietary and lifestyle changes made.

Variability of Results:

The aim of this book is to aid individuals in enhancing their overall health through informed dietary choices. However, it is acknowledged that individual results can vary significantly. Factors such as genetics, lifestyle, medical history, and program adherence play a crucial role in the effectiveness of the strategies discussed.

Priority of Professional Medical Advice:

In instances where the advice provided in this book conflicts with recommendations given by a reader's doctor or healthcare provider, it is imperative that the individual adhere to the professional guidance of their healthcare provider. The information in this book is not intended to replace or supersede any advice or prescriptions provided by medical professionals.

Medication and Treatment:

Readers are cautioned against making any changes to their medication or treatment plans without first consulting with their healthcare provider. Stopping medication or altering treatment regimens without professional guidance can have serious health consequences.

Liability Limitation:

The author(s) and publisher of "2024 Glycemic Index & Load Diet for Diabetes" shall not be held liable for any direct, indirect, incidental, consequential, or any other damages that may arise from the use, or misuse, of the information provided. Readers assume full responsibility for any actions taken based on the information contained in this book and agree to use discretion and seek professional advice when necessary.

CONTENTS

Introduction   ix

THE LOW GLYCEMIC INDEX &
LOAD DIET FOR DIABETES

Part I
UNDERSTANDING DIABETES: A
COMPREHENSIVE GUIDE

1. Diabetes, Insulin and Insulin Resistance   5
2. Understanding Type 1 and Type 2 Differences   10
3. Diabetes Complications and Risks   18
4. Diabetes Tests & Diagnosis   24
5. Hypoglycemia, a Feared Complication of Diabetes   27
6. The ABCDE of diabetes   32

Part II
KNOWING WHAT'S IN THE FOOD YOU EAT

7. Carbohydrate Essentials: What You Need to Know   39
8. Protein — the building blocks of life   44
9. Lipids — Essential Macronutrients for Health   49
10. Essential Micronutrients In Diabetes Diet   54

Part III
THE LOW GL DIABETES DIET: A SUSTAINABLE
STRATEGY FOR ENHANCED BLOOD SUGAR
MANAGEMENT

11. The Low-GL Diet: Understanding the Concept and   61
    Reaping the Benefits
12. The 15 Core Principles   72
13. Common Questions & Answers   77

Part IV

DIETARY GUIDELINES AND MEAL PLANNING
PRINCIPLES

14. Meal Planning Guidelines – The Three-Tiered Approach   85
to Diabetes Meal Planning
15. Dietary Guidelines and the Structured Approach of the   88
Low GL Diabetes Diet
16. Macronutrient distribution for your Low GL Diabetes Diet   92
17. The plate Method   96
18. Crafting a One-Day Meal Plan   99

Part V

LOW GL DIABETES DIET FOOD LISTS

19. The Vegetables Diabetes-friendly Food Lists   109
20. The Fruits Diabetes-friendly Food Lists   122
21. The Grains Diabetes-friendly Food Lists   133
22. The Dairy and Plant-Based Alternatives Diabetes-friendly 139
Food Lists
23. Protein DiabetesDiabetes-friendly Food Lists   147

THE GI, GL & NET CARB COUNTER

1. Introduction to the Glycemic Index and Glycemic Load   157
Counter
2. Breads and Baked Products   160
3. Beans & Lentils   170
4. Beverages   177
5. Dairy products   184
6. Dairy Alternatives — Plant-based Options   191
7. Dressings & Oils   196
8. Fruits   201
9. Fruit Products   211
10. Grains, Cereals, Pasta & Rice   220
11. Herbs and Spices   230
12. Nuts & seeds   234
13. Vegetables & Vegetable Products   237

Bibliography/References   247

Health and Nutrition Websites   251
About the Author   253

INTRODUCTION

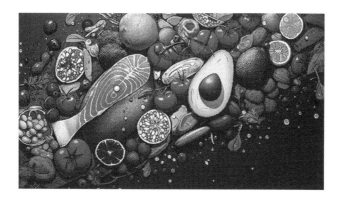

Success in diet management, particularly for diabetes, relies significantly on how you manage carbohydrate intake. Although current Centers for Disease Control and Prevention (CDC) guidelines suggest that about 45-50% of our daily caloric intake should come from carbohydrates, the real challenge in diabetes management transcends these percentages. It involves understanding how different carbohydrates affect blood sugar levels and integrating this knowledge into daily meal planning—a strategy proven to substantially improve glucose control and blood markers.

I developed this awareness over 27 years, not as a patient, but as a pharmacist working closely with those affected by diabetes, witnessing the burdens and poor outcomes of uncontrolled diabetes due to adherence to unfriendly dietary patterns. My extensive experience has allowed me to observe various trajectories of diabetes control, ranging from poor to excellent. Seeing the complexities involved in integrating carbohydrate management into a diabetes diet firsthand has shown me that this aspect of diabetes management is significantly more intricate than in other conditions, such as hypertension or kidney disease. In those conditions, the focus generally lies on restricting specific micronutrients like sodium, phosphorus, potassium, and protein. Unlike these simpler dietary modifications, carbohydrates present unique challenges; their diverse structures and functions affect blood sugar levels in non-uniform ways. This variability highlights the necessity of a sophisticated dietary approach that utilizes tools like the Glycemic Index (GI) and Glycemic Load (GL). These tools help differentiate between foods that stabilize blood sugar levels and those that lead to significant fluctuations, thus supporting more effective diabetes management.

The Low glycemic Index & Load Diabetes Diet presented in this book offers a comprehensive solution that transcends simple carbohydrate management by embracing the broader principles of healthy eating recommended by the 2020-2025 Dietary Guidelines for Americans. This diet emphasizes the consumption of nutrient-rich, whole, and minimally processed foods, incorporating healthy fats such as polyunsaturated and monounsaturated fats. It addresses the core issues of unhealthy eating patterns by substantially reducing the intake of ultra-processed foods, sugary drinks, advanced glycation end-products (AGEs), and foods high in sodium, saturated, and trans fats. By doing so, the Low-GL Diabetes Diet mirrors the essential elements of a balanced and nutritious diet, proving to be an effective, science-backed strategy for managing diabetes and enhancing overall health.

Developed in the early 1980s by Dr. David Jenkins, the Glycemic Index (GI) is a scientific scale designed to aid those with diabetes by showing how different carbohydrates impact blood sugar levels. While the GI was groundbreaking, its guidelines were initially vague and could lead to overconsumption, potentially undermining diabetes management. To refine this approach, Harvard researchers introduced the Glycemic Load (GL) concept in 1997. The GL enhances the GI by considering both the type of carbohydrate and the quantity consumed. Each GL unit corresponds to the effect of consuming one gram of glucose, providing a scale with direct physiological relevance.

With this advancement, the Glycemic Load has become critical in managing diabetes, offering substantial benefits for dietary planning and metabolic health. It classifies foods based on their impact on blood sugar and their carbohydrate content per standard serving size, helping individuals maintain their daily carbohydrate intake within the recommended 45%-50% of total calories. The application of GL principles in meal planning is straightforward, proven, and easily integrated into daily life, enabling better blood glucose control, preventing or halting complications, and improving overall health.

Here, we encapsulate the crucial insights gleaned from current research, emphasizing significant findings:

- **Better Blood Sugar Control**: Eating foods with a low Glycemic Load (GL) helps people with diabetes control their blood sugar levels after meals. This means fewer sudden spikes in blood sugar, making diabetes easier to manage.
- **Less Inflammation**: Foods with a lower GL can reduce inflammation in the body. Inflammation is linked to various health problems and complications, so this is a big plus for overall health.
- **Improved Metabolic Health**: Lowering the GL in your diet can also aid maintain your blood sugar, insulin, and fat levels in a healthier range over time. This supports your body's metabolism both now and in the future.

- **Benefits for Diabetic Conditions**: Some fruits, like grapes, which have low-GL, are particularly good for reducing high blood sugar and supporting the health of cells that produce insulin, partly thanks to their natural compounds called polyphenols.
- **Significant Health Improvements**: Diets low in GL have been shown to help lower long-term blood sugar levels and improve cholesterol, body weight, and blood pressure. This kind of diet, when combined with medications, can significantly enhance overall health and diabetes management.

THE PRACTICAL LOW-GL DIET PLAN FOR DIABETES MANAGEMENT

Managing diabetes effectively requires a carefully considered diet to stabilize blood sugar levels. This book serves as a practical guide to the low glycemic Index and Load Diabetes Diet, blending the principles of GI and GL with Mediterranean and balanced diet elements. This approach improves glycemic control, prevents complications, and may even delay the progression of existing conditions.

'The Low-GL Diabetes Diet' is grounded in rigorous scientific research and enhanced by real-life experiences. It summarizes extensive meta-analyses and successful case studies, addressing common challenges in diabetes management and integrating stories from individuals who have successfully managed their diabetes. These stories explore both the dietary changes and the emotional challenges of long-term diabetes management.

Supported by a vast bibliography, this guide offers a blend of empirical data and personal narratives, providing a scientifically sound yet deeply personal approach to diabetes management. The book covers both basic and advanced dietary strategies:

- **Basic Level:** Features straightforward, immediately applicable tools such as diabetes-friendly food lists, standardized carb servings, the plate method, and 15 fundamental principles for meal planning.
- **Advanced Stage:** Expands on the initial tools with a comprehensive glycemic index, glycemic load, and net carb counter, offering detailed nutritional values for managing diabetes effectively.

Many users have seen significant blood sugar improvements, with some achieving remission. This book highlights the practical and theoretical underpinnings of the Low-GL Diabetes Diet, enhancing management and reducing the risk of complications.

THE LOW GLYCEMIC INDEX & LOAD DIET FOR DIABETES

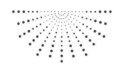

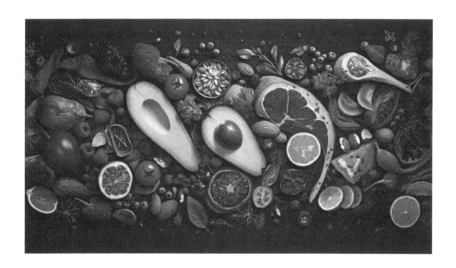

PART I
UNDERSTANDING DIABETES:
A COMPREHENSIVE GUIDE

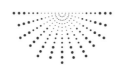

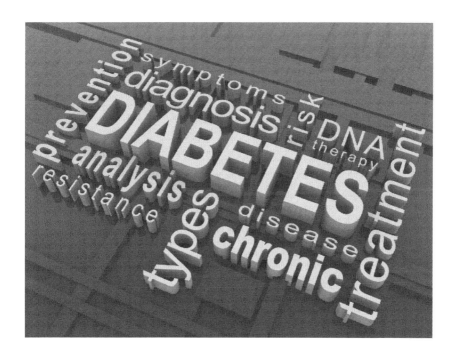

1

DIABETES, INSULIN AND INSULIN RESISTANCE

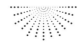

INSULIN RESISTANCE

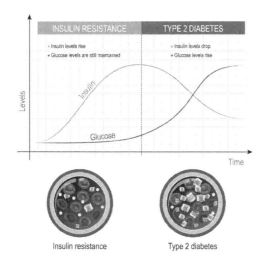

Insulin resistance   Type 2 diabetes

UNDERSTANDING INSULIN IN DIABETES MANAGEMENT

When diagnosed with diabetes or when managing the condition, the term 'insulin' often comes up. But what exactly is insulin? Is it a medication, a treatment, or a natural hormone? How does it relate to diabetes, including concepts like 'insulin resistance' and 'insulin sensitivity'? This chapter provides clear explanations and actionable advice.

Understanding Insulin

Insulin is a crucial hormone for human health and is one of the most studied due to its vital role in metabolic processes. It is produced by the beta cells within the islets of Langerhans in the pancreas. As a protein hormone, insulin is essential for regulating glucose levels in the blood and cell metabolism, facilitating the cellular uptake of glucose for energy production.

Insulin's primary function is to maintain the body's energy balance by regulating blood glucose levels. After food intake, carbohydrates are broken down into glucose, which enters the bloodstream. Elevated glucose levels prompt the pancreas to release insulin, which enables the entry of glucose into the body's cells. There, it is used for energy or stored for future use, thereby regulating the body's metabolic processes.

The infographic below provides a schematic representation of how insulin facilitates glucose entry into cells. It outlines four key steps:

1. **Presence of Insulin and Glucose**: Insulin and glucose are available outside the cell, with insulin receptors highlighted on the cell surface.
2. **Insulin Binds to Receptors**: Insulin binds to its receptors, initiating a signal that activates glucose channels.
3. **Glucose Entry into the Cell**: The channels open, allowing glucose to enter the cell.

4. **Glucose Utilization**: Glucose inside the cell is used for energy, illustrating effective cellular uptake.

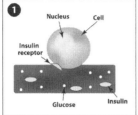
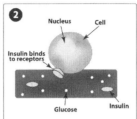
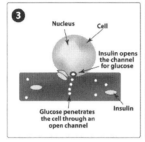
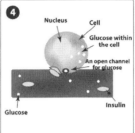

Insulin Action Mechanism Detailed: The infographic "How Does Insulin Work" visually encapsulates the details of insulin's action within the body. Insulin acts like a biological key that unlocks cell membranes, allowing glucose to enter cells from the bloodstream. This process is crucial for preserving energy balance and proper cellular function. Insulin attachs to an insulin receptor on the cell membrane, which triggers the glucose channels to transition from a closed to an open state, facilitating glucose's entry into the cell, where it is utilized for energy.

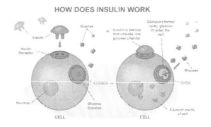

HOW DOES INSULIN WORK

Optimal Blood Sugar Levels: Insulin plays a pivotal role in regulating blood sugar within a healthy range, ideally between 60-100 mg/dL when fasting and under 140 mg/dL after meals. These levels are essential for the body's optimal functioning and help avoid the extremes of hyperglycemia and hypoglycemia. Proper insulin function ensures that glucose is efficiently stored and utilized, maintaining energy balance and metabolic stability. Inadequately controlled blood sugar levels can lead to significant complications, resulting in irreversible damage to organs and tissues.

INSULIN AND DIABETES

Diabetes arises from disruptions in insulin's regulatory function. In Type 1 Diabetes (T1D), the body stops producing insulin, necessitating lifelong insulin therapy to manage blood glucose levels. This is depicted in the infographic below, showing the mechanism of T1D, where the pancreas produces no insulin, leading to heightened blood sugar levels as glucose cannot enter the cells.

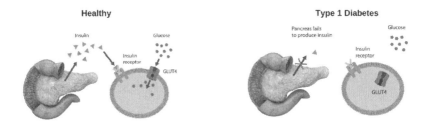

In contrast, Type 2 Diabetes (T2D) typically begins with insulin resistance, where cells lose their ability to respond appropriately to insulin despite its presence. Over time, the pancreas struggles to keep up with the increased demand for insulin, resulting in progressively worse glucose control. To improve insulin sensitivity, initial management strategies for T2D focus on lifestyle changes (e.g., diet and exercise). As the condition advances, medications that enhance the body's response to insulin may be required, and eventually, some individuals might also need insulin therapy. This progression is visualized in the infographic below, illustrating how the pancreas still produces insulin but at insufficient levels, and muscle cells do not effectively utilize glucose due to insulin resistance.

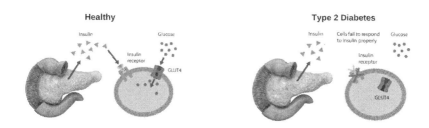

2

UNDERSTANDING TYPE 1 AND TYPE 2 DIFFERENCES

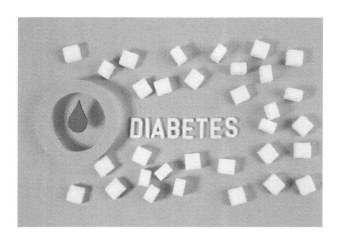

A BRIEF HISTORY OF DIABETES

Diabetes mellitus is a common metabolic condition characterized by chronic hyperglycemia due to disruption in insulin secretion, insulin action, or both. Without appropriate treatment, it can lead to life-threatening complications. Diabetes is categorized into two main types: Type 1 diabetes (T1D), which is insulin-dependent, and Type 2 diabetes (T2D), which is non-insulin-dependent.

Recognition of diabetes dates back to ancient civilizations, including Egypt, Greece, China, and India. These cultures identified three main symptoms: excessive urination (polyuria), sugar in the urine (glycosuria), and intense thirst (polydipsia), all contributing to gradual body wasting, highlighting the disease's catabolic nature.

One of the earliest detailed descriptions of diabetes was provided by Aretaeus of Cappadocia, a physician in the 2nd century AD, who described it as "the melting down of flesh and limbs into urine." Centuries later, Islamic physician Abu Bakr Muhammad Al-Razi, known as Rhazes, documented diabetes in his works, using a diagnostic method involving observing whether ants were attracted to a patient's urine—a sign of elevated glucose levels.

The term "diabetes mellitus," meaning "honey-sweet," was coined in the 1600s by Thomas Willis, reflecting the sweet-smelling urine characteristic of the disease due to excess sugar. Significant advancements in understanding diabetes occurred in the early 20th century with Frederick Banting and Charles Best's discovery of insulin in 1923, revolutionizing diabetes treatment, especially T1D. In 1936, Sir Harold Percival Himsworth differentiated Type 1 from Type 2 diabetes by identifying insulin resistance as a key factor in T2D.

Following the discovery of insulin, further refinements included the development of longer-acting insulins and insulin analogs. The advent of home blood glucose monitoring in the 1970s enabled patients to manage their blood glucose levels actively, improving individual care. Recent decades have seen the introduction of medications that improve insulin sensitivity, reduce hepatic glucose production, and enhance glucose excretion, offering more comprehensive management strategies for T2D. Technological advances, such as continuous glucose monitoring systems and insulin pumps, have automated insulin delivery, easing the daily burden of disease management. Research into the genetic foundations of T1D and the development of immune therapy is paving the way for potential preventive treatments.

BLOOD GLUCOSE REGULATION - HEALTHY INDIVIDUALS

Regulating blood glucose is vital for health and well-being. In individuals with normal pancreatic function, this regulation is finely tuned. After consuming foods, particularly carbohydrates, the digestive system metabolizes them into glucose, which enters the bloodstream. This rise in blood glucose triggers the pancreas to secrete insulin, a hormone that enables glucose uptake by cells throughout the body for energy. Any glucose not immediately needed is stored in the liver as glycogen.

During fasting periods, such as overnight or between meals, the pancreas releases glucagon. Glucagon signals the liver to degrade stored glycogen and release glucose back into the bloodstream, maintaining stable blood sugar levels. The balance between insulin and glucagon ensures a steady supply of glucose to the body's cells while preventing levels from becoming too high or too low.

UNDERSTANDING TYPE 1 DIABETES

TYPE 1 DIABETES

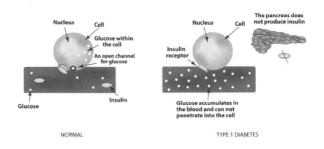

NORMAL   TYPE 1 DIABETES

Type 1 diabetes is an intricate autoimmune disorder where immune system attacks pancreatic beta cells, destroying them and preventing the pancreas from producing insulin. This process is irreversible, causing blood sugar to build up due to the lack of insulin. Daily insulin injections and careful dietary management are crucial for survival and minimizing severe health complications. T1D occur at any age but is most commonly diagnosed in children and young adults. Unlike T2D, T1D is not primarily caused by lifestyle factors, although genetic predisposition and environmental factors, such as viral infections, can influence its development.

Type 1 Diabetes Pancreas Functioning:

1. After eating, individuals with T1D experience a rise in blood glucose due to the absence of insulin secretion following the autoimmune destruction of beta cells.
2. The lack of insulin prevents glucose from entering cells, causing persistent hyperglycemia.
3. The liver, unaware of the high glucose levels due to the absence of insulin, releases more glucose, adding to the already high blood sugar.
4. Energy production is compromised without insulin; external insulin is required for glucose management.
5. People with T1D rely on lifelong insulin therapy as their bodies cannot naturally regulate blood sugar levels.

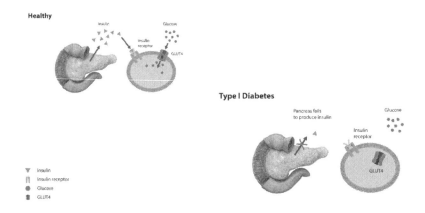

Pancreas Anatomy in Type 1 Diabetes:

- The pancreas may appear smaller due to the significant loss of beta cells.
- Insulitis, or inflammation of the islets, is typically observed, marked by immune cell infiltration and beta-cell destruction.
- The anatomical changes lead to a marked deficiency in insulin production.

Advancements in Treatment: In 2016, the FDA approved the artificial pancreas, a significant development in T1D management. These devices mimic the function of a healthy pancreas by automatically monitoring blood glucose levels and administering insulin as needed, providing a more stable and responsive treatment method.

Risk Factors for Type 1 Diabetes:

- **Family History:** Higher likelihood with a close relative who has the disease.
- **Ethnicity:** Caucasians in the U.S. have a higher incidence.
- **Age:** Commonly diagnosed in children and adolescents, but can occur at any age.

- **Viral Infections:** Certain viruses can trigger an autoimmune response.
- **Vitamin D Deficiency:** Essential for immune regulation.

Symptoms of Type 1 Diabetes:

- Frequent thirst and urination
- Intense hunger
- Diabetic ketoacidosis (DKA)
- Unexplained weight loss
- Blurred vision
- Abdominal pain
- Frequent infections
- Fatigue

Recognizing these symptoms early is crucial for timely diagnosis and management of T1D to prevent complications and stabilize blood sugar levels.

UNDERSTANDING TYPE 2 DIABETES

TYPE 2 DIABETES

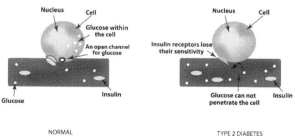

NORMAL   TYPE 2 DIABETES

ype 2 diabetes (T2D) is a prevalent metabolic illness resulting from a combination of insulin resistance and pancreatic beta-cell dysfunction. Initially, the pancreas responds to insulin resistance by increasing insulin production. However, over time, this response may become inadequate. T2D accounts for the majority of diabetes cases and can occur at any age, though it's most common after forty. With rising obesity rates and poor dietary choices, T2D increasingly affects younger populations.

Type 2 Diabetes Pancreas Functioning:

1. The body's cells resist insulin, hampering glucose absorption.
2. The pancreas produces more insulin to overcome resistance, but this can lead to beta-cell fatigue.
3. As pancreatic output falters, glucose accumulates in the bloodstream.
4. The liver may inappropriately release more glucose, exacerbating the condition.
5. Persistent hyperglycemia necessitates medical intervention to manage blood sugar levels.

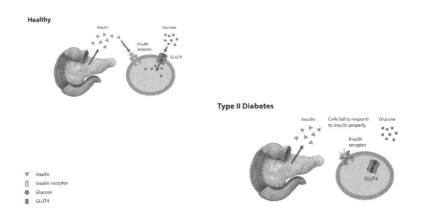

Pancreas Anatomy in Type 2 Diabetes:

- The pancreas may vary in size; some may have an enlarged pancreas due to initial beta-cell overactivity.
- Beta cells show signs of dysfunction and may decrease in number.
- Amyloid deposition within the islets of Langerhans is common, disrupting insulin secretion.

Risk Factors for Type 2 Diabetes:

- Overweight and obesity
- Family history
- Ethnic background
- Age
- High blood pressure
- Polycystic ovary syndrome (PCOS)
- Vitamin D deficiency

Symptoms of Type 2 Diabetes:

- Increased thirst and urination
- Weight loss
- Fatigue
- Blurred vision
- Slow healing
- Recurrent infections

These symptoms and risk factors underscore the importance of early detection and proactive management of T2D to prevent complications and maintain health.

3

DIABETES COMPLICATIONS AND RISKS

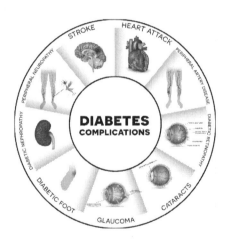

WHY WE EMPHASIZE THE IMPORTANCE OF UNDERSTANDING COMPLICATIONS?

The rationale behind dedicating an entire chapter to complications, rather than merely listing them, is grounded in the severe and potentially life-altering stakes involved. Diabetes complications can be devastating, significantly affecting quality of life and posing severe health risks. Awareness of these complications alone is insufficient; it's equally crucial to understand the controllable risk factors to mitigate their impact. This approach goes beyond the basics of diabetes risk factors, delving into the risk factors for complications themselves —an aspect often overlooked in discussions about diabetes.

FROM MANAGEABLE CONDITION TO SEVERE THREAT

When managed with diligent care, including diet, lifestyle modifications, and medication, diabetes can be a manageable condition, imposing minimal restrictions on life. However, absent vigilant management, diabetes morphs into a menacing presence capable of inflicting extensive damage across the body. The spectrum of microvascular to macrovascular complications, including neuropathy, nephropathy, retinopathy, cardiovascular diseases, stroke, and peripheral vascular disease, paints a vivid picture of potential outcomes. The progression to peripheral vascular disease, with its dire consequences of non-healing wounds, gangrene, and possible amputation, starkly illustrates the severity of neglect.

GRASPING THE GRAVITY OF COMPLICATIONS

Recognizing the severe nature of these complications is essential for treating diabetes management as a non-negotiable priority. Understanding the risk factors for diabetes-related complications empowers you to act decisively against them. This real-world observation, drawn from countless patient experiences, underscores the stark reality that neglecting rigorous diabetes management, including risk factor mitigation, dietary intervention, and lifestyle modifications, can lead to severe complications. Many find themselves trapped in a cycle of progressively increasing medication adjustments, unaware of the critical need to halt the disease's progression early on. As diabetes progresses, the rate at which complications intensify can escalate rapidly, underscoring the necessity for early and assertive management strategies. The relationship between diabetes and diabetic kidney disease (DKD) vividly illustrates this point, serving as a sobering reminder of the importance of prevention and the imperative for intensified efforts if complications arise.

TRANSITIONING TO THE BROADER IMPLICATIONS OF DIABETES COMPLICATIONS

Diabetes is a leading cause of significant health complications and mortality in the United States, with a profound impact on healthcare costs. The severity of diabetes complications, which can be both devastating and life-threatening, often stems from chronic high blood sugar compounded by other conditions such as hypertension. Although the initial mechanisms—where excess glucose in the bloodstream inflicts damage on the body's vessels and organs—may seem straightforward, the progression of these complications is inherently complex and multifaceted.

Taking chronic kidney disease (CKD) as a prime example, we see a condition deeply feared in the context of diabetes. CKD arises when elevated glucose levels strain the kidneys' filtering capacity to its limits, initiating a series of damages to the nephrons, the kidneys' microscopic filtering units. Diabetic kidney disease (DKD), as identified by Mogensen in the 1980s, starts with microalbuminuria and, without intervention, can advance to macroalbuminuria, signaling a deterioration in kidney function.

As diabetes progresses, its interaction with CKD becomes increasingly complex. Beyond the early stages, where the direct impact of high glucose levels harms the kidneys, the aggravation of CKD further complicates diabetes, weaving a dense web of mutual exacerbation. This intricate and non-linear progression highlights the critical importance of proactive diabetes management. It's not just about managing diabetes in isolation but understanding and addressing the interplay with conditions like CKD to prevent a cascade of complications, emphasizing the necessity of a comprehensive approach to care that considers the wide-reaching implications of this chronic disease.

EXPLORING THE COMPLEXITIES OF DIABETES AND ITS COMPLICATIONS

Understanding the intricate relationship between diabetes and its complications is essential. Both Type 2 Diabetes (T2D) and Type 1 Diabetes (T1D) present unique challenges but share many complications that can have profound effects on the body's organs and systems. By delving deeper into the specific complications associated with T2D and T1D, we aim to highlight the extensive range of issues that can arise, underlining the critical need for comprehensive management strategies.

Common Complications Across Diabetes Types:

- **Cardiovascular Disease:** Diabetes exacerbates the risk of cardiovascular issues by promoting atherosclerosis, where chronic high blood sugar levels cause inflammation and injury to blood vessels. This leads to plaque buildup, increasing the risk of heart disease, heart attacks, and strokes.
- **Neuropathy:** Long-term high blood sugar can damage nerves, causing neuropathy. Symptoms include numbness, tingling, pain, and weakness, primarily affecting the extremities. This can drastically reduce quality of life, making everyday activities challenging.
- **Nephropathy:** The kidneys' vulnerability to diabetes can lead to diabetic nephropathy, progressing to chronic kidney disease (CKD). This complication may require dialysis or a kidney transplant, highlighting the importance of early detection and management.
- **Ophthalmic Complications:** Diabetes can damage the retina's blood vessels, causing diabetic retinopathy. Untreated,

it can develop into severe vision impairment or blindness, underscoring the importance of regular eye exams.

- **Peripheral Vascular Disease:** Impaired blood flow, especially to the limbs, can result from diabetes, increasing the risk of ulcers, non-healing wounds, and potentially leading to amputation in severe cases of infection or gangrene.
- **Dental Health Issues:** Diabetes is linked to deteriorating oral health, including gum diseases, cavities, and increased plaque formation. Regular dental care is vital to prevent serious dental issues.
- **Immune System Weakening:** Diabetes can compromise the immune system, increasing susceptibility to infections and slowing wound healing, necessitating vigilant care and prevention strategies.
- **Mental Health Concerns:** Managing diabetes's chronic nature can be mentally taxing, potentially leading to anxiety and depression. This underscores the importance of addressing the psychological aspects of diabetes care and ensuring patients receive support for their mental and physical health.

T1D-SPECIFIC CHALLENGES:

While T1D and T2D share many complications, the autoimmune nature and typically earlier onset of T1D require additional vigilance. Individuals with T1D may face a higher or more rapid progression of these complications, making early intervention and continuous management paramount. The distinct challenges of T1D, including its unpredictable blood sugar variations and the constant need for insulin management, demand a tailored approach to complication prevention and treatment.

Expanding the Scope of Diabetes Management:

Expanding our understanding of the spectrum of complications associated with diabetes can help us better appreciate the necessity for a comprehensive approach to diabetes care. This includes regular monitoring for early signs of complications, personalized treatment plans that address both T1D and T2D's unique challenges, and comprehensive support that encompasses the physical, dental, and mental health of individuals with diabetes.

4

DIABETES TESTS & DIAGNOSIS

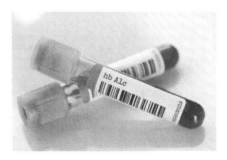

The diagnosis of type 1 and type 2 diabetes typically involves assessing blood sugar levels through various tests, enabling healthcare professionals to make an accurate assessment. Common tests for diagnosing and monitoring diabetes include:

FASTING BLOOD SUGAR TEST (FPG)

This test evaluates blood glucose levels following an overnight fast, typically lasting eight hours or more.

Interpreting FPG results:

- Normal: An FPG level ≤ 99 mg/dL.
- Prediabetes: An FPG level between 100 mg/dL (5.6 mmol/L) and 125 mg/dL (7 mmol/L), indicating a higher risk of developing diabetes.
- Diabetes: An FPG level ≥ 126 mg/dL.

HBA1C TEST

This test measures the percentage of hemoglobin in red blood cells coated with glucose, reflecting the average blood sugar level over the past two to three months.

Interpreting A1C results:

- Normal: A1C level under 5.7%.
- Prediabetes: A1C level between 5.7% and 6.4%, indicating a higher chance of developing diabetes.
- Diabetes: A1C level ≥ 6.5%.

ORAL GLUCOSE TOLERANCE TEST (OGTT)

During the OGTT, the individual consumes a sugary solution, and blood sugar levels are measured two hours later.

Interpreting OGTT results:

- Normal: A 2-hour glucose level ≤ 140 mg/dL.
- Prediabetes: A 2-hour glucose level between 140 mg/dL and 199 mg/dL, indicating a higher risk of diabetes.
- Diabetes: A 2-hour glucose level ≥ 200 mg/dL.

RANDOM BLOOD SUGAR TEST (RPG)

The random blood sugar test is used to diagnose diabetes when symptoms are present, allowing testing without fasting.

Interpreting RPG results:

- Diabetes: An RPG blood glucose level $\geq$ 200 mg/dL.

C-PEPTIDE TEST

This test measures C-peptide, a byproduct of insulin production, to gauge insulin levels in the body. It helps distinguish between type 1 and type 2 diabetes.

- Type 1 Diabetes: Low C-peptide levels indicate reduced insulin production.
- Type 2 Diabetes: Elevated or normal C-peptide levels suggest insulin resistance with relatively preserved insulin secretion.

Upon diagnosis, diabetes management focuses on attaining and sustaining optimal blood sugar levels, preventing complications, and improving overall health and wellness.

5

HYPOGLYCEMIA, A FEARED COMPLICATION OF DIABETES

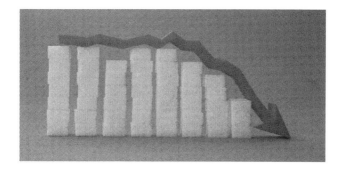

Hypoglycemia, defined as an abnormally low plasma glucose concentration, is a critical issue in diabetes management, especially for individuals relying on insulin therapy, sulfonylureas, or glinides. This condition poses a significant health risk, particularly to individuals with type 1 diabetes, though it can also impact those with type 2 diabetes. An international study showed that 80% of individuals with type 1 diabetes and nearly 50% of those with type 2 diabetes experienced at least one episode of hypoglycemia over a four-week period.

Certain diabetes medications, such as dipeptidyl peptidase-4 inhibitors, metformin, glucagon-like peptide-1 receptor agonists, thiazolidinediones, and sodium-glucose cotransporter-2 inhibitors, generally present a lower risk of hypoglycemia. However, insulin and insulin secretagogues significantly elevate this risk due to their direct effect on increasing insulin production or release. This necessitates meticulous management and monitoring.

The American Diabetes Association (ADA) and the European Medicines Agency define hypoglycemia as "any abnormally low plasma glucose concentration that exposes the subject to potential harm," with a threshold plasma glucose value of <70 mg/dL (<3.9 mmol/L).

WHY IS HYPOGLYCEMIA DANGEROUS?

Glucose is the brain's primary energy source. An acute interruption of glucose supply can result in a rapid decline in cognitive function, leading to symptoms ranging from confusion and abnormal behavior to severe outcomes like coma and death. Without prompt treatment, hypoglycemia can impair brain function, causing irreversible harm.

Hypoglycemia's danger lies in its immediate impact on cognitive and physical abilities, potential to cause accidents and injuries, and risk of long-term neurological damage. Recurrent episodes can lead to hypoglycemia unawareness, where the body's normal response to low blood glucose becomes blunted, delaying recognition and treatment.

Given these risks, diabetes management strategies must proactively prevent hypoglycemia, including balancing medication, diet, and exercise, utilizing continuous glucose monitoring (CGM) technology, and educating patients to recognize and respond to early signs of hypoglycemia.

SYMPTOMS OF HYPOGLYCEMIA

Symptoms typically manifest when blood glucose drops to 70 mg/dL or lower. These symptoms serve as alerts to correct low blood sugar.

Mild-to-moderate hypoglycemia symptoms:

- Rapid or irregular heartbeat
- Shaking
- Sweating
- Anxiety or irritability
- Dizziness or lightheadedness
- Hunger

Severe hypoglycemia symptoms:

- Loss of consciousness
- Confusion or disorientation
- Concentration difficulties
- Behavioral changes, such as nervousness or irritability
- Convulsions or seizures
- Coma

Understanding these symptoms is essential for people with diabetes to promptly address hypoglycemia and prevent dangerous consequences.

DIAGNOSING HYPOGLYCEMIA

Hypoglycemia is diagnosed by recognizing its symptoms and confirming low blood glucose levels. Episodes are classified into three levels of severity to guide intervention:

- **Level 1 hypoglycemia:** Plasma glucose levels below 70 mg/dL but above 54 mg/dL, signaling the need for intervention.
- **Level 2 hypoglycemia:** Plasma glucose levels below 54 mg/dL, indicating a significant drop that requires immediate action.
- **Level 3 hypoglycemia:** Severe episodes where mental or physical capabilities are compromised, necessitating help from others.

CAUSES OF LOW BLOOD GLUCOSE IN INDIVIDUALS WITH DIABETES

Factors leading to low blood sugar include:

- **Over-medication:** Taking too much insulin or medicines that stimulate insulin release.
- **Dietary Mismanagement:** Insufficient carbohydrate consumption, meal delays, or skipping meals, especially when taking insulin or certain drugs.
- **Fasting:** Especially risky while on insulin or glucose-lowering drugs.
- **Excessive Exercise:** Physical activity with low carbohydrate intake may cause sudden insulin drops.
- **Weather Conditions:** Hot and humid weather can enhance insulin absorption, raising hypoglycemia risk.
- **Alcohol Consumption:** Especially with heavy drinking and certain medications, the liver may not release enough glycogen to maintain blood sugar levels.

HYPOGLYCEMIA UNAWARENESS

This condition occurs when a person does not notice hypoglycemia symptoms. Regular blood sugar checks or continuous glucose monitoring (CGM) devices may be necessary to detect and address low levels promptly.

PREVENTION AND TREATMENT OF HYPOGLYCEMIA

Prevention strategies for diabetes patients:

- **Regular Glucose Checks:** Consistently monitor glucose levels as recommended.
- **Consistent Meal Times:** Eat regularly scheduled, nutritionally balanced meals.

- **Proper Medication Adherence:** Follow prescribed insulin or diabetes medication dosages strictly.
- **Exercise Caution:** Adjust carbohydrate intake and insulin doses based on physical activity.

TREATMENT FOR HYPOGLYCEMIA

Immediate action is crucial when dealing with hypoglycemia.

The 15-15 Rule: For blood sugar levels between 55 and 69 mg/dL, eat 15 to 20 grams of fast-acting carbohydrates and recheck sugar levels after 15 minutes. Repeat as needed and eat a sustaining meal or snack afterward.

Options for 15 to 20 grams of fast-acting carbohydrates:

- 3 teaspoons of sugar, honey, or corn syrup
- 3 glucose tablets
- ½ cup (4 oz) of fruit juice or soda
- A slice of bread, a small banana, a medium apple, regular yogurt, or 20 grapes
- ½ cup of cooked couscous or pasta
- 1 cup (8 oz) of milk

SEVERE HYPOGLYCEMIA MANAGEMENT

In severe cases, others must administer glucagon, available in nasal spray and injection forms, to rapidly increase blood glucose levels. Ensure family, friends, and coworkers know how to spot severe hypoglycemia, use glucagon, and know where it is kept.

6

THE ABCDE OF DIABETES

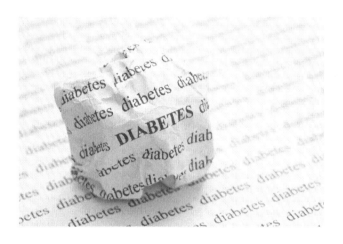

THE ABCDE OF DIABETES MANAGEMENT: A COMPREHENSIVE FRAMEWORK

The ABCDE of diabetes management provides a structured and holistic framework to enhance the effectiveness of diabetes care and improve overall health outcomes. This approach emphasizes critical aspects of managing diabetes and promotes a comprehensive strategy to boost well-being across various facets of life.

BLOOD MARKERS MONITORING AND ITS IMPACT

Monitoring key blood markers is pivotal in managing diabetes and preventing complications. Persistent high blood sugar levels can cause severe hypertension, affecting nearly half of those diagnosed with type 2 diabetes. This condition can constrict blood vessels, adversely impacting vital organs and potentially leading to significant health complications. Additionally, diabetes can drastically alter the lipid profile in the bloodstream, raising the likelihood of cardiovascular diseases. Regular and vigilant monitoring of these markers is crucial to averting such detrimental outcomes.

THE ROLE OF LIFESTYLE ADJUSTMENTS IN DIABETES MANAGEMENT

Effective diabetes management encompasses more than just dietary adjustments; it also involves making targeted lifestyle changes. This comprehensive approach emphasizes the importance of regular physical activity, proper hydration, and sufficient sleep, all of which are crucial for better blood sugar control and enhanced insulin sensitivity. Regular physical activity and adequate sleep help stabilize blood sugar levels and decrease the risks associated with diabetes-related complications.

Strategic Framework: The ABCDE of Diabetes Management

- **A1C (HbA1c) Test:** The A1C test is an essential indicator of long-term glucose control, reflecting average blood sugar levels over the past two to three months. For most adults with diabetes, it is advised to keep the A1C level under 7% to minimize the risk of complications like neuropathy, retinopathy, and cardiovascular diseases. However, A1C targets can be individualized based on factors such as age, duration of diabetes, presence of complications, and overall health. Stricter targets (below 6.5%) may be set for younger individuals or those without significant heart disease, while less stringent targets (such as 8% or slightly higher) might be appropriate for older adults or those with complex health issues.

- **Blood Pressure Management:** Controlling blood pressure is crucial for individuals with diabetes, as hypertension significantly elevates the risk of cardiovascular diseases. Current guidelines generally recommend a target blood pressure of less than 130/80 mm Hg for most people with diabetes. This target can be achieved through lifestyle modifications such as diet, exercise, and, if necessary, pharmacological treatments. Targets may be personalized based on individual risk factors and co-existing medical conditions.

- **Cholesterol Management:** Dyslipidemia, characterized by high LDL cholesterol, high triglycerides, and low HDL cholesterol, is prevalent among those with diabetes and raises the risk of cardiovascular complications. Monitoring lipid levels is essential, and treatment should be tailored to individual needs. This often involves dietary adjustments, physical activity, and potentially lipid-lowering medications. Treatment goals typically include lowering LDL cholesterol to less than 100 mg/dL, with adjustments based on overall health and specific cardiovascular risk profiles.

- **Diet and Nutrition:** A low glycemic impact balanced diet is vital in managing diabetes and preventing its complications. It's essential to balance nutrient intake, include fiber-rich foods, and monitor carbohydrate consumption. Dietary patterns such as the low glycemic load diet, the Mediterranean diet, DASH, and plant-based diets are beneficial for those with diabetes.

- **Exercise and Physical Activity:** Regular exercise is crucial for managing diabetes and enhancing overall health. It improves insulin sensitivity, aids in weight management, and lowers the risk of heart disease. Health guidelines advocate at least 150 minutes of moderate-to-intense aerobic activity each week, as well as muscle-strengthening exercises.

Personalized Management Considerations:

- **Timely Medications:** Adhering to prescribed diabetes medications is vital for maintaining optimal glucose levels.
- **Low GI and GL Food Choices:** Opting for foods with a low glycemic impact helps regulate blood sugar levels effectively. A varied diet, including fruits, vegetables, grains, proteins, and dairy, while limiting unhealthy fats and processed foods, is advisable.
- **Physical Activity:** Regular exercise helps maintain normal glucose levels. Aim for at least 30 minutes of moderate-intensity activity on most days.
- **Regular Glucose Monitoring:** For those with type 1 diabetes and insulin-dependent individuals, monitoring blood sugar levels is crucial. A glucose meter or CGM (continuous glucose monitoring) helps keep glucose levels within the target range.

PART II
KNOWING WHAT'S IN THE FOOD YOU EAT

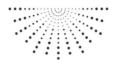

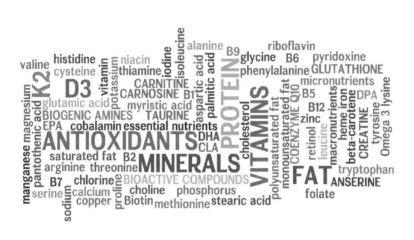

7

CARBOHYDRATE ESSENTIALS: WHAT YOU NEED TO KNOW

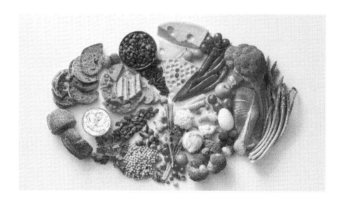

Managing diabetes effectively involves more than just restricting carbohydrates; it requires understanding how different types of carbohydrates impact blood sugar levels. Over the past 25 years, I've noted a common misconception that carbohydrates must be drastically reduced due to their impact on blood sugar. However, extreme restrictions are neither practical nor beneficial since carbohydrates are essential energy sources that our bodies need.

Balancing Carbohydrate Intake

The High-Fat, Low-Carb (HFLC) diet, which limits carbohydrate intake to as low as 15% of daily calories, aims to manage blood sugar and help in weight loss. Despite its popularity, this diet doesn't consistently deliver results for everyone and can lead to health issues such as heart disease, gout, and kidney strain due to higher protein and fat intake.

EVOLUTION OF DIABETES MANAGEMENT APPROACHES

Diabetes management has evolved significantly, from using exchange lists in the early 2000s to adopting the Glycemic Index (GI) and Glycemic Load (GL) models. These models reflect a deeper understanding of how carbohydrates affect blood sugar stability.

IMPORTANCE OF DIETARY FIBER

Incorporating sufficient dietary fiber is essential to manage diabetes and prevent complications. A daily intake of 25 to 30 grams of fiber stabilizes blood sugar levels, supports heart health, reduces stroke and hypertension risks, and maintains gastrointestinal health.

Recent Insights on Dietary Fiber in Diabetes Management

- **Type 2 Diabetes (T2DM) Management:** High dietary fiber intake decreases T2DM risk and aids in prevention and management.
- **Gut Health and T2DM:** Dietary fiber positively affects gut bacteria, crucial for managing T2DM and boosting immunity.
- **Fiber Supplementation (STAR Survey):** Physicians recommend fiber supplements for T2DM, noting improvements in blood sugar levels, weight management, and cholesterol levels.
- **Viscous Soluble Fiber:** This significantly lowers blood sugar and cholesterol levels in T2DM.
- **Gestational Diabetes:** Fiber supplements improve glucose

levels, HbA1c, and lipid profiles, enhancing pregnancy outcomes.

Determining the Right Amount of Fiber

For individuals with diabetes, it is recommended to eat 20 to 35 grams of fiber daily from sources like raw vegetables and unprocessed grains, aiming for 14-16 grams of fiber per 1,000 calories. Ensure at least half of the grain intake is from whole grains. High-fiber carbohydrates (over 5 grams per serving) include legumes, whole grain breads, cereals, and fruits and vegetables. Gradually increase fiber intake to avoid gastrointestinal issues.

Balancing carbohydrate intake is crucial, with recommendations suggesting 45-50% of total daily calories from carbohydrates. This approach emphasizes high-quality, fiber-rich carbohydrates for effective diabetes management and metabolic health.

CARBOHYDRATES WITHIN THE LOW-GL DIABETES DIET

A common question among individuals with diabetes is, "What can I eat to maintain my blood sugar levels within the therapeutic target?"

The Glycemic Index (GI) categorizes foods based on their impact on blood glucose levels. Considering the quantity of carbohydrates consumed, we can determine a food's Glycemic Load (GL), providing insight into its physiological effect on blood sugar.

Carbohydrate Classification: Simple vs. Complex

Carbohydrates are divided based on their molecular structure into:

- **Complex Carbohydrates:** Found in unprocessed foods like vegetables, fruits, legumes, and whole grains. They digest slowly, stabilizing blood sugar levels.
- **Simple Carbohydrates:** Found in processed foods, refined sugars, and snacks, leading to quick spikes in blood glucose

levels. Frequent consumption is tied to health risks such as metabolic syndrome, T2DM, and obesity.

Carbohydrates are further divided into three main types:

- **Sugars:** Simple carbohydrates comprise short-chain molecules, including fructose, glucose, sucrose, and galactose. They are rapidly metabolized, causing abrupt blood sugar spikes.
- **Starches:** Complex carbohydrates that break down into glucose during digestion, providing a steadier energy release.
- **Fibers:** Indigestible carbohydrates that maintain digestive health and significantly affect blood sugar control.

NAVIGATING CARBOHYDRATES IN A DIABETES DIET

The standard advice for managing diabetes includes prioritizing complex carbohydrates and minimizing simple carbohydrates and added sugars. However, not all simple carbohydrates impact health equally. For instance, fruits contain simple sugars but also offer vital vitamins and nutrients. Due to their nutrient density and fiber content, whole fruits can moderate their effect on blood sugar levels, unlike processed foods and sugary drinks.

The Glycemic Index and Glycemic Load

The Glycemic Index and Glycemic Load offer a sophisticated framework for meal planning. Applying GI and GL values helps differentiate between beneficial and detrimental foods for diabetes management. This approach guides dietary decisions to regulate crucial hormones, including insulin, leptin, ghrelin, cortisol, and peptide YY.

Diabetes Macronutrient Distribution

Understanding "diabetes macronutrient distribution" empowers you to tailor your diet to meet your health objectives. Adopting the correct dietary strategy can lead to successful diabetes management. The low-GL Diabetes Diet equips you with the necessary tools and knowledge to manage your condition effectively and live a healthier life.

By following these guidelines, individuals with diabetes can make informed dietary choices, effectively manage their blood sugar levels, and improve overall health.

8

PROTEIN — THE BUILDING BLOCKS OF LIFE

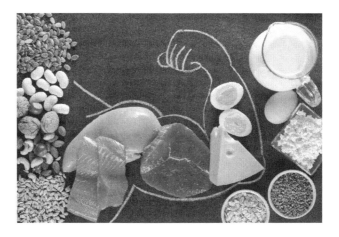

Proteins, alongside carbohydrates and fats, are foundational elements in our diet and vital for maintaining health. They provide the body with amino acids and small peptides, crucial for constructing cellular structures and synthesizing essential metabolites, including purines, pyrimidines, and neurotransmitters.

Unlike other macronutrients, proteins play unique roles in the body. They constitute about three-fourths of the dry matter in most human tissues, except for bone and fat. These large molecules are essential for virtually all vital functions, serving as catalysts for chemical reactions, regulating gene expression, and forming the structure of cells and muscles.

STRUCTURAL AND FUNCTIONAL ROLES OF PROTEINS

Proteins are critical for building and maintaining the body's physical framework. They are integral to every cell, tissue, and organ, including muscles, bones, skin, and hair, providing necessary structure and supporting overall physical functionality.

Proteins also regulate the immune system, facilitate neurotransmission, and act as enzymes, hormones, and receptors that enable cell communication. This dual role as both building blocks and active biological molecules underscores their indispensable nature in maintaining health and supporting essential bodily operations.

THE CRITICAL ROLE OF AMINO ACIDS

Amino acids—the building blocks of proteins, are organic compounds that play diverse roles in the body. They act as precursors for hormones and neurotransmitters, which are essential for communication and physiological regulation. For example, tryptophan is a precursor for the serotonin, a critical neurotransmitter involved in depression and mood and sleep regualtion.

Proteins are indispensable in tissue synthesis and repair, influencing muscle growth and wound healing. They also play an important role in enzyme production, speeding up metabolic processes from digestion to DNA replication. Additionally, proteins form antibodies that are essential for immune response.

The 9 Essential Amino Acids

Our diets need to provide nine essential amino acids—histidine, isoleucine, leucine, lysine, methionine, phenylalanine, threonine, tryptophan, and valine—as the body cannot synthesize them. These amino acids are needed for tissue repair, immune response, and hormone synthesis.

These essential amino acids are found in both animal-based and plant-based foods. Meats, dairy products, and eggs provide all nine essential amino acids. Plant-based foods like nuts, beans, and lentils also contain these amino acids but may need to be combined to reach a complete amino acid profile.

The Importance of Protein in the Diet

Unlike fats and carbohydrates, proteins lack a specialized storage form, emphasizing the need for regular protein consumption. This is especially important during growth, recovery from injury, or increased physical activity. Proteins regulate critical physiological processes, such as hormone activity, enzymatic reactions, and immune responses.

Proteins also have a higher thermogenic effect than lipids and carbo-hydrates, playing a significant role in metabolic regulation and body composition. They help regulate energy expenditure and metabolic rate, contribute to weight management, enhance satiety, and reduce excess calorie consumption.

PROTEIN INTAKE GUIDELINES

The Recommended Dietary Allowance (RDA) for protein, set at 0.8 grams per kilogram of body weight for adults, represents the minimum amount needed to avoid deficiency. However, this amount may not be optimal for improving health and facilitating muscle growth.

Optimal Protein Intake Across Different Groups

- **Normal Weight Individuals with No Chronic Kidney Disease (CKD):** The RDA of 0.8 grams per kilogram of body weight is a baseline to prevent deficiency. Higher intakes (1.2-2.0 grams per kilogram) may benefit those who are physically active, older adults, or athletes.

- **Individuals with Overweight or Obesity and Normal Kidney Function:** Higher protein intake (1.2-2.0 grams per kilogram) can aid weight loss by promoting satiety and boosting metabolic rate.
- **Individuals with Diabetes and Early-Stage CKD:** Limiting protein intake to 0.8–1.0 grams per kilogram per day helps manage kidney disease progression.
- **Individuals with Advanced CKD:** Protein intake should be reduced to about 0.8 grams per kilogram per day to prevent further kidney function decline.

DIABETES AND PROTEIN CHOICES

Individuals with diabetes should avoid ultra-processed meats and high-sodium meat products. Nutrient-dense, plant-based proteins offer fiber and antioxidants beneficial for overall health. However, plant-based diets require careful planning to avoid deficiencies in zinc, vitamin B12, calcium, and certain essential amino acids.

UNDERSTANDING COLLAGEN: THE BODY'S BUILDING BLOCK

What is Collagen?

Collagen, making up about 27-30% of total protein in the human body, is essential for tissue integrity, elasticity, and regeneration. It supports ligaments, tendons, skin, hair, nails, intervertebral discs, bones, and connective tissues.

Main Types of Collagen:

- **Type I:** Found in skin, tendons, and bones, maintaining structural integrity.

- **Type II:** Found in cartilage and bones, supporting connective tissues.
- **Type III:** Found in muscles, blood vessels, the uterus, and intestines, providing support and elasticity.

Aging and Collagen Synthesis:

Collagen synthesis decreases with age, starting around age 30 and accelerating after age 50. This reduction can lead to muscle stiffness, joint aging, wrinkles, loss of skin tone, slower wound healing, and increased fatigue.

Collagen for Diabetes:

Collagen supplementation can offer multiple health benefits, including improved skin quality, healthier joints, stabilized blood sugar levels, and supported cardiovascular health. It may also benefit intestinal health, which is crucial for those with diabetes.

Optimal Collagen Intake:

While there is no consensus on the exact amount, ensuring adequate collagen in the diet provides significant health advantages. For individuals with diabetes, collagen can enhance skin condition, ease joint pain, aid blood sugar control, and support heart health.

9

LIPIDS — ESSENTIAL MACRONUTRIENTS FOR HEALTH

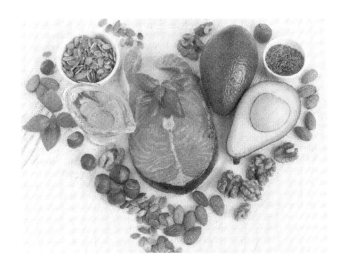

Dietary fats, or lipids, are essential macronutrients crucial for various physiological functions and serve as the body's main source of stored energy. Found in foods like fats, oils, meats, dairy products, and certain plants, they are primarily consumed as triglycerides. Lipids not only store energy but also contribute to cellular structure and function, regulate body temperature, and protect organs. One gram of lipid provides 9 kcal of energy, more than double the calories provided by carbohydrates or proteins, which supply 4 kcal per gram.

WHY IS FAT ESSENTIAL FOR YOUR HEALTH?

Lipids are fundamental for several reasons:

- **Nutrient Absorption:** Fats facilitate the absorption of fat-soluble vitamins (A, D, E, and K), vital for vision, bone health, antioxidant protection, and blood clotting.
- **Hormone Production:** Fats are crucial in synthesizing hormones that regulate growth, metabolism, and reproductive health.
- **Regulation of Inflammation and Immunity:** Omega-3 fatty acids help reduce inflammation and support immune function.
- **Cell Health Maintenance:** Fats are key components of cell membranes, affecting cell integrity and function, including skin and hair health.

CLASSIFICATION OF DIETARY FATS AND THEIR INFLUENCE ON HEALTH

There are four primary types of dietary fats:

- **Saturated Fat:** Saturated fat, a type of lipid found naturally in animal products and certain plant oils, is linked to heart disease. Moderation is recommended, especially for individuals with diabetes, CKD (Chronic Kidney Disease), or an increased risk of cardiovascular disease.
- **Trans Fat:** Chemically altered fats to enhance food shelf life, linked to heart disease and inflammation. Should be minimized in the diet.
- **Monounsaturated Fats (MUFAs):** Found in olive oil,

avocados, and certain nuts, these fats promote heart health and blood sugar control.

- **Polyunsaturated Fats (PUFAs):** Includes omega-3 and omega-6 fatty acids found in fish, flaxseeds, and specific oils. Essential for reducing inflammation and supporting heart and brain health.

UNDERSTANDING CHOLESTEROL: ITS ROLE AND TYPES

Cholesterol is a vital fat-like substance present in every cell, essential for several biological functions, including:

- **Vitamin D Synthesis**
- **Steroid and Sex Hormone Production:** Such as cortisol, aldosterone, testosterone, estrogens, and progesterone.
- **Formation of Bile Salts:** Crucial for digesting and absorbing fat-soluble vitamins.

Types of Cholesterol:

- **LDL Cholesterol (Low-Density Lipoprotein):** Known as "bad" cholesterol, high levels can lead to plaque accumulation in arteries, increasing heart disease risk.
- **HDL Cholesterol (High-Density Lipoprotein):** Known as "good" cholesterol, it aids in moving cholesterol from the blood to the liver, where it is excreted in the form of bile, which helps decrease the risk of heart disease.

Cholesterol Synthesis and Dietary Impact

The liver the majority of the body's cholesterol, while dietary cholesterol contributes less significantly. More than 85% of blood cholesterol is synthesized endogenously. Thus, dietary cholesterol has a minor impact on blood cholesterol levels.

The Health Implications of Cholesterol Imbalance

An imbalance, particularly high LDL cholesterol levels, can lead to conditions like hypercholesterolemia, significantly increasing the risk of cardiovascular diseases. Thus, it is vital for people with diabetes and cardiovascular disease to manage their cholesterol levels to mitigate associated risks.

Recommended Fat Types for Optimal Health in Diabetes

To manage diabetes and prevent complications, focus on natural, unprocessed fat sources, especially those high in monounsaturated and omega-3 fatty acids. These fats help manage cholesterol levels, reduce inflammation, and support cardiovascular health.

Healthy Fat Sources:

- **Avocado and Avocado Oil:** Rich in monounsaturated fats, beneficial for heart health and cholesterol management.
- **Fatty Fish (Sardines, Anchovies, Salmon):** Excellent sources of omega-3, known for reducing inflammation and supporting heart health.
- **Olives and Olive Oil:** Packed with MUFAs and antioxidants, olive oil helps stabilize blood sugar levels.
- **Nuts and Nut Oils (Macadamias, Almonds, Brazil Nuts, Hazelnuts, Pecans):** Provide a balanced blend of monounsaturated and polyunsaturated fats.
- **Flaxseeds and Flaxseed Oil:** Good sources of alpha-linolenic acid (ALA), an omega-3 with anti-inflammatory properties.
- **Walnuts and Walnut Oil:** Rich in omega-3 fatty acids, improving endothelial function and cardiovascular health.
- **Chia Seeds:** Packed with omega-3, fiber, and antioxidants, supporting heart health and blood glucose management.
- **Sunflower Seeds and Sunflower Oil:** Provide vitamin E and healthy fats, to be consumed in moderation due to higher omega-6 content.

- **Extra Virgin Olive Oil:** Abundant in antioxidants and monounsaturated fats, beneficial for heart health and managing diabetes and CKD.

By focusing on these healthy fats, individuals with diabetes can better manage their condition and support overall health.

10

ESSENTIAL MICRONUTRIENTS IN DIABETES DIET

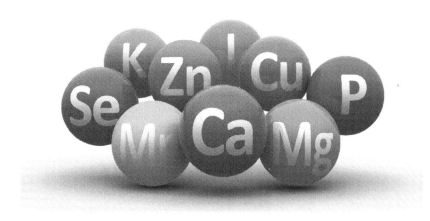

Micronutrients, including essential minerals and vitamins, are crucial for human health, regulating vital physiological functions throughout life. Despite being needed in small amounts, they play a significant role in maintaining overall well-being. Insufficient intake of one or more of these nutrients can lead to severe health outcomes, especially for people with diabetes, hypertension, heart disease, and early-stage Chronic Kidney Disease (CKD).

Significance of Micronutrients in Metabolic Functions

Micronutrients are vital for numerous metabolic reactions and tissue functions. Deficiencies can lead to various symptoms, including:

- Fatigue and sleep disturbances
- Mood changes and irritability
- Cognitive impairments
- Increased stress levels
- Paleness
- Digestive issues
- Chronic headaches
- Muscle tension
- Heart palpitations

Micronutrient deficiencies are particularly concerning for individuals with diabetes, as they can impact bodily functions and contribute to the progression of the disease and its complications. Common micronutrient deficiencies in people with diabetes include:

- **Iron:** Essential for the making of hemoglobin, which transports oxygen in the blood and is vital for preventing anemia.
- **Vitamin D:** Crucial for bone health, immune function, and regulating calcium absorption.
- **Iodine:** Necessary for the thyroid hormones production , which regulate metabolism.
- **Calcium:** Key for maintaining bone structure, muscle function, and nerve function.
- **Vitamins B12 and B9 (Folate):** Important for neurological function, DNA formation, and red blood cell production.
- **Vitamin A:** Vital for vision, immune health, and skin integrity.
- **Zinc:** Important for immune function, wound healing, and DNA synthesis.

- **Magnesium:** Involved in over 350 biochemical reactions, including energy production, nerve function, and muscle relaxation.
- **Vitamin C:** Important for immune function, skin health, and antioxidant protection.
- **Vitamin E:** A potent antioxidant with roles in cell protection and immune support.
- **Selenium:** Critical for metabolism, thyroid function, and antioxidant properties.

MICRONUTRIENTS IN DIABETES MANAGEMENT

Managing diabetes benefits from careful attention to micronutrient levels. Emerging research suggests that certain micronutrients may have therapeutic benefits in managing Type 2 Diabetes Mellitus (T2DM):

- **Vitamin D:** May improve glycemic control and reduce the risk of diabetes-related complications by enhancing insulin sensitivity and reducing inflammation.
- **Vitamin K:** May aid in improving vascular health and insulin sensitivity, potentially reducing inflammation and diabetes-related complications.
- **Magnesium:** Plays a role in glucose metabolism, with adequate levels associated with better blood sugar control and a lower risk of T2DM.
- **Chromium:** Believed to enhance insulin sensitivity. Caution is advised when taking chromium supplements with diabetes medications, as they can lower blood sugar levels and increase the risk of hypoglycemia, especially when used with insulin, metformin, or other medications that improve insulin sensitivity or increase beta-cell insulin release.

By understanding the role of these micronutrients, individuals managing diabetes can take proactive steps to maintain adequate levels and support overall health.

PART III
THE LOW GL DIABETES DIET:
A SUSTAINABLE STRATEGY
FOR ENHANCED BLOOD
SUGAR MANAGEMENT

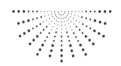

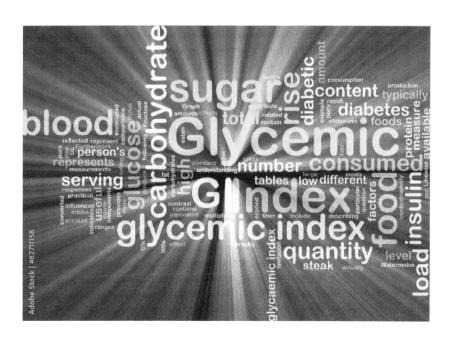

11

THE LOW-GL DIET: UNDERSTANDING THE CONCEPT AND REAPING THE BENEFITS

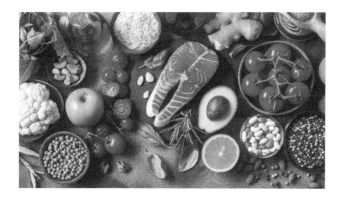

Effective diabetes management traditionally focuses on optimizing markers like glycated hemoglobin (HbA1c), fasting plasma glucose (FPG), and postprandial glucose (PPG), as recommended by the American Diabetes Association. The low glycemic index & load (GL) diet transcends its original function of merely categorizing foods based on their glycemic impact. It has evolved into a comprehensive dietary strategy that emphasizes the quality and quantity of carbohydrates, advocating for a balanced and nutritious eating pattern.

This dietary approach, as promoted in this book, goes beyond just assessing the glycemic impact. It includes practical elements tailored explicitly for diabetes management, such as portion control with a standard serving size of 15 grams of carbohydrates, as per the CDC guidelines. It aligns with the 2020-2025 Dietary Guidelines for Americans, covering aspects that indirectly affect blood sugar levels.

Type 2 diabetes is characterized by persistent hyperglycemia and insulin resistance, leading to complications if unmanaged. The Low-GL Diabetes Diet targets these issues by moderating blood glucose spikes and reversing insulin resistance through diet quality improvement, weight loss, intermittent fasting, and the inclusion of dietary elements like Extra Virgin Olive Oil (EVOO). This straightforward, evidence-based approach provides crucial insights for effective carbohydrate management and improved blood glucose control.

The benefits of adhering to the Low-GL Diabetes Diet principles are significant compared to merely counting carbohydrates. Followers of this diet generally experience more stable blood sugar levels, lower A1C levels, and improved lipid profiles. In contrast, those focusing solely on carbohydrate counting tend to report poorer diabetes control and less favorable health outcomes.

Since the 2000s, I have advocated for considering both the glycemic index value and carbohydrate content of foods, a practice supported by many endocrinologists. To aid this, I have compiled a comprehensive list of common foods, detailing their glycemic index, portion size, carbohydrate content, and glycemic load. This resource has helped thousands of patients stabilize their blood sugar and improve their A1C by choosing lower GI foods.

UNDERSTANDING THE GLYCEMIC INDEX: POSTPRANDIAL BLOOD GLUCOSE RESPONSES

Postprandial Blood Glucose Responses: The Foundation of the GI Concept

Postprandial responses, which have been studied extensively in the fields of physiology, endocrinology, and biochemistry, are vital for understanding how our body reacts to different foods. Significant milestones such as the discovery of secretin by William M. Bayliss and Ernest H. Starling in 1902, and insulin by Frederick Banting and Charles Best in 1921, have been pivotal in advancing our knowledge about how blood sugar is regulated after meals, especially in the context of diabetes management.

Immediate Response to Food Intake:

- **Carbohydrate Absorption:** When we consume food, the carbohydrates present are metabolized into glucose and absorbed into the bloodstream. This process leads to an increase in blood glucose levels, the extent of which is influenced by the type of carbohydrates consumed, as well as the meal's fiber, fat, and protein content.

The Body's Insulin Response:

- **Insulin Release and Function:** The pancreas secretes insulin in response to increased glucose levels. This hormone plays a crucial role in permitting glucose uptake by cells for energy use or storage, thereby helping to decrease blood glucose levels.

THE GLYCEMIC INDEX AS A DIETARY TOOL:

The GI concept's importance was underscored by historical discoveries like secretin in 1902 by William M. Bayliss and Ernest H. Starling, and insulin in 1921 by Frederick Banting and Charles Best. These discoveries have substantially advanced our understanding of blood sugar regulation post-meal, particularly in diabetes management.

Developed in 1981 by Dr. David Jenkins and his team at the University of Toronto, the GI measures how carbohydrate-rich foods impact blood glucose levels compared to pure glucose. This tool aids in managing blood sugar levels and refining dietary choices.

Factors Influencing Glycemic Responses:

- **Starch Composition and Properties:** Factors like digestibility and the amylose/amylopectin ratio influence glycemic responses, along with changes due to cooking (gelatinization) and cooling (retrogradation).
- **Dietary Fiber:** The type and amount of fiber can significantly affect glycemic responses.
- **Types of Sugar:** Variations in sugars impact blood glucose levels differently.
- **Additional Influential Factors:** These include insulin response, protein content, food processing techniques, particle size, fat content, acidity, storage conditions, and harvest time.

GLYCEMIC INDEX CATEGORIZATION:

Foods are categorized into three groups based on their post-meal blood glucose impact:

- **High-GI (GI ≥ 70):** These foods are quickly metabolized and absorbed, inducing rapid spikes in blood glucose and insulin levels.
- **Medium-GI (GI between 56 and 69):** These foods have a moderate impact on blood glucose.

- **Low-GI (GI ≤ 55):** These foods are metabolized and absorbed slowly, resulting in a gradual increase in blood glucose levels.

This classification helps individuals understand and manage how different foods affect their blood sugar levels, supporting better diabetes control and overall health management.

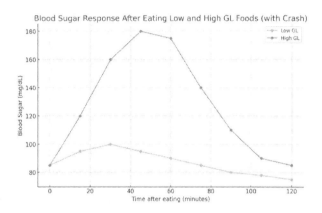

To clarify this concept, let's examine the examples of an apple and a ripe banana, both calibrated to have the same net carbohydrate content. By comparing these two fruits, which have different glycemic index values despite similar carbohydrate content, we can illustrate how the GI concept elucidates the physiological impacts of various foods on blood sugar levels.

Example 1: Apple

• **Food:** Apple (1 medium, approximately 183g)

• **Net Carbohydrates:** 21 grams

• **Glycemic Index (GI):** 36

A medium-sized apple weighing around 183 grams contains 21 grams of net carbohydrates and has a GI of 36. A low GI value indicates that the apple will have a relatively minimal effect on blood sugar levels compared to pure glucose.

To determine how many grams of pure glucose would have a similar effect on blood sugar as this apple, we use the following formula:

$$\text{Equivalent glucose amount} = \left(\frac{\text{Net carbohydrates}}{100}\right) \times \text{GI}$$

Substituting in the values:

$$\text{Equivalent glucose amount} = \left(\frac{21 \text{ grams}}{100}\right) \times 36$$

$$\text{Equivalent glucose amount} \approx 7.56 \text{ grams}$$

Equivalent glucose amount≈7.56 grams

- Thus, **consuming a medium-sized apple similarly affects blood sugar as consuming approximately 7.56 grams of pure glucose.**

Example 2: Ripe Banana

- Food: Banana (1 small, approximately 85g)
- Net Carbohydrates: 21 grams
- Glycemic Index: 75

In this example, a small ripe banana with the same net carbohydrate content as the apple (21 grams) has a GI of 75, which is significantly higher. This suggests a greater impact on blood sugar levels. Calculating the equivalent glucose effect:

$$\text{Equivalent glucose amount} = \left(\frac{21 \text{ grams}}{100}\right) \times 75$$

$$\text{Equivalent glucose amount} \approx 15.75 \text{ grams}$$

- Thus, **consuming a small banana similarly affects blood sugar as consuming approximately 15.75 grams of pure glucose.**

These two examples demonstrate how the Glycemic Index (GI) can be used to categorize foods based on their impact on blood sugar, allowing for more precise comparisons. Even though both the apple and banana have similar net carbohydrate content, the apple's lower GI value means it has a lesser impact on blood sugar levels.

LIMITATIONS OF THE GLYCEMIC INDEX CONCEPT

While the glycemic index provides valuable insights into how foods affect blood sugar, it has several limitations:

- **Portion Sizes Not Accounted For:** GI measures the impact of a standard amount of carbohydrate in foods, not considering the quantity consumed. The Glycemic Load (GL) complements GI by factoring in serving size to reflect a food's effect on blood sugar more accurately.
- **Food Preparation and Combination Effects:** The GI of a food can vary based on its preparation method. For example, pasta cooked al dente typically has a lower GI compared to overcooked pasta. Additionally, combining foods, such as incorporating fats or proteins, can modify the glycemic response to a carbohydrate-rich meal.
- **Neglect of Nutrient Content:** GI does not reflect the nutritional richness of foods. Some high-GI foods are nutrient-dense, while some low-GI foods offer little

nutritional value. Relying solely on GI could mislead people about the healthiness of their food choices.

- **Limited Scope for Non-Carbohydrate Foods:** Foods without carbohydrates, like pure meats and oils, lack a GI value, which can lead to confusion when planning a balanced diet.
- **Inconsistencies in Food GI Values:** Variations in GI can occur even within the same type of food due to differences in ripeness, processing, and brand, leading to inconsistencies and potential confusion for those trying to adhere to GI guidelines.

These limitations emphasize the need for a balanced approach. While GI can be beneficial for diet management, relying solely on it can lead to overconsumption of low-GI foods, resulting in overeating, potential nutritional imbalances, and inconsistent blood sugar control.

THE LOW-GL DIABETES DIET: BALANCING GLYCEMIC IMPACT

The Low-GL Diabetes Diet enhances the Glycemic Index (GI) by incorporating the Glycemic Load (GL) concept, which assesses both the quality and quantity of foods consumed. This method aligns with the latest nutritional guidelines, such as the 9th edition of Dietary Guidelines for Americans, and integrates principles from the Mediterranean diet to promote a balanced dietary regimen. This approach aims to rectify the shortcomings of the GI system, which can lead to nutritional inconsistencies.

For instance, the GI system would permit consuming large amounts of mango (GI of 54) while discouraging even small portions of watermelon (GI of 72) due to its higher GI. This could lead to consuming significantly more carbohydrates from mangoes, despite the lower GI, potentially harming both diabetics and non-diabetics alike. Additionally, the GI approach may inadvertently favor lower-quality foods with low GI values, such as artificially produced margarine with trans fats, illustrating the system's limitations.

The Low-GL Diabetes Diet addresses these issues by applying the GL concept, which considers both the glycemic index and the carbohydrate content of a standard serving, providing a more comprehensive assessment of food's impact on blood sugar levels. Developed by Harvard researchers, the GL metric offers a more precise tool for diabetes management by correlating the blood sugar response to actual food intake rather than just categorizing foods based on their GI.

The GL system helps manage portion sizes effectively, reducing the risk of carbohydrate overconsumption and the associated blood sugar spikes. It supports a diverse and nutritious diet by promoting appropriate portion sizes and minimizing excessive carbohydrate intake risks.

GLYCEMIC LOAD RANKINGS:

- **Low-GL (10 or less):** These foods have a minimal impact on blood sugar, making them excellent choices for maintaining stable glucose levels throughout the day.
- **Medium GL (11 to 19):** Foods in this category moderately affect blood sugar. They can be occasionally included in the diet, considering the total carbohydrate intake and timing relative to activity levels.
- **High GL (20 or more):** Foods with a high GL significantly influence blood sugar levels and should be consumed sparingly, if at all, particularly by those managing strict blood sugar control.

By leveraging the GL system, the Low-GL Diabetes Diet overcomes the limitations of the GI approach, offering a more effective and balanced way to manage diabetes through diet.

ADDITIONAL CONSIDERATIONS:

Glycemic Load of Combined Meals: The glycemic load (GL) of a meal is determined by summing the GLs of each component. Even if individual foods have low-GL values, their combination can lead to a higher total GL, potentially impacting blood sugar levels.

Recommendations on Added Sugars: Authoritative organizations like the CDC and the ADA (American Diabetes Association) recommend that individuals with diabetes limit added sugar intake to no more than 10% of total daily calories, equating to a maximum of 50 grams or 50 GL per day.

Impact of Food Processing: The GL of food can increase with processing. Foods that are highly processed often have higher GL values compared to those that are whole and minimally processed.

Balancing Carbohydrates with Proteins and Fats: To reduce the glycemic impact, combine carbohydrates with proteins and healthy fats. This approach helps manage glycemic load by providing sustained energy and fullness.

Timing of Meals and Snacks: Distributing meals and snacks evenly throughout the day helps maintain stable blood sugar levels and prevents spikes. Each meal should include a balanced mix of carbohydrates, proteins, and fats.

Physical Activity: Regular exercise leads to numerous health benefits, such as enhanced insulin sensitivity and better blood sugar regulation.

WATERMELON: A CASE STUDY IN GLYCEMIC INDEX AND LOAD

Watermelon serves as an informative example for understanding the glycemic index and load concepts. Despite a high GI of 72, watermelon has a low-GL of approximately 6 due to its modest carbohydrate content. A standard serving of 120 grams, about two thin slices, contains about 11.5 grams of carbohydrates and 9 grams of natural sugars, which is less than the recommended serving of 15 grams of carbohydrates. Thus, its GL is categorized as low, indicating that watermelon is a viable option for blood sugar management.

Postprandial Impact of Watermelon:

Upon consuming a 150-gram serving of diced watermelon, the body absorbs the simple sugars (sucrose, fructose, and glucose) along with 11.5 grams of carbohydrates. Despite its high GI, indicating rapid sugar release into the bloodstream, the actual impact on blood sugar is moderate due to the low-GL. This is further influenced by its minimal fiber (0.6 grams per serving) and almost no fat content.

Comparative Dietary Implications:

Eating watermelon, with its low-GL, contrasts significantly with high-GI and high-GL foods, which can cause more pronounced blood sugar spikes. Thus, understanding and utilizing the GL of foods like watermelon supports informed dietary choices, allowing for the inclusion of various fruits while managing glycemic control effectively.

THE 15 CORE PRINCIPLES

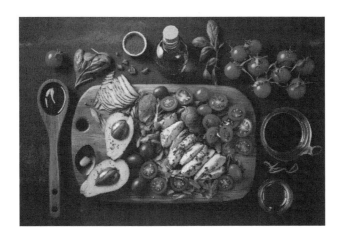

THE LOW-GL DIABETES DIET: A PRACTICAL GUIDE TO MANAGING DIABETES

The Low-GL Diabetes Diet is built on 15 principles that simplify adopting healthy eating habits. These principles are particularly beneficial and practical for individuals managing diabetes. They also address challenges like the risks from processed foods, the effects of high-glycemic-index foods, and the dangers of excessive sugar and sodium intake.

These practical and comprehensive guidelines enhance diabetes care and overall well-being. They are designed to be user-friendly, suitable for flashcards, reminder cards, or quick reference notes, based on real-life patient experiences that highlight the need for straightforward dietary guidance.

Key Principles Include:

Principle 1: Prioritize Low Glycemic Load Foods

Focus on foods that aid in weight management, enhance blood sugar control, and support overall health. Emphasize whole, minimally processed foods in line with the latest dietary guidelines.

Principle 2: Increase Olive Oil Consumption

Incorporate extra-virgin olive oil (EVOO) for its monounsaturated fats, which can enhance cholesterol levels, reduce inflammation, and lower heart disease risk. Aim for at least four tablespoons daily to maximize its anti-diabetic and antioxidant effects.

Principle 3: Limit Added Sugars

Reduce intake of sugars that appear under various names like corn syrup and fructose. These hidden sugars, especially prevalent in processed foods, can substantially affect blood sugar levels and contribute to metabolic issues related to diabetes.

Principle 4: Reduce Sodium Intake

Manage sodium consumption to combat the heightened risk of hypertension and other severe diabetes-related complications. The Dietary Guidelines for Americans (DGA) recommend restricting sodium to less than 2,300 mg per day, emphasizing the importance for individuals with both diabetes and hypertension.

Principle 5: Incorporate Polyphenol-Rich Foods

Incorporating polyphenol-rich foods is crucial in the Low GL Diabetes Diet. Polyphenols, potent antioxidants present in many plants, can reduce inflammation, enhance insulin utilization, and lower the risk of chronic health issues. Choose foods like berries, dark chocolate, green tea, red wine, extra-virgin olive oil, and apples, cherries, spinach, and kale to increase dietary polyphenols. These foods support overall health and aid in managing weight and diabetes by improving insulin efficiency and reducing inflammation.

Principle 6: Choose Flavonoid-Rich Foods

Flavonoids, another group of antioxidants, are beneficial for reducing inflammation and enhancing insulin utilization, which is crucial for preventing chronic diseases. Rich sources include berries, apples, onions, blueberries, cherries, spinach, kale, dark chocolate beverages like green and black teas, and red wine. Including these foods in your diet helps manage blood sugar, protect the brain, potentially reduce cancer risk, and maintain healthy blood vessels.

Principle 7: Opt for Healthy Fats

Healthy fats are vital in the low-GL diabetes Diet, providing necessary energy and aiding nutrient absorption. Focus on a balanced intake of monounsaturated and polyunsaturated fats, which support cardiovascular health and reduce inflammation. Restrict saturated fats to less than 10% of daily caloric intake, as recommended by the DGA.

Principle 8: Boost Omega-3 Fatty Acid Intake

Increasing omega-3 fatty acids and reducing omega-6 fats is essential, aiming for an omega-6/omega-3 ratio between 4:1 and 3:1. Omega-3s minimize heart disease risk and support overall health, while high omega-6 levels can lead to inflammation. Increase your omega-3 intake with nuts, seeds, and fatty fish like salmon, sardines, and mackerel.

Principle 9: Add Anti-Inflammatory Spices

Enhance meals with anti-inflammatory spices such as turmeric, garlic, ginger, cinnamon, and cumin, and use fresh herbs to replace or reduce salt. While beneficial, spices and herbs should complement a balanced diet that includes whole grains, vegetables, pulses, fruits, lean proteins, and healthy fats.

Principle 10: Avoid Foods with Artificial Trans Fats

Eliminate artificial trans fats linked to heart disease and other health issues. These fats are found in many processed foods, like baked goods and fried items. Choose products free of trans fats by reading labels and inquiring about cooking oils in restaurants.

Principle 11: Stay Hydrated with Water

Staying hydrated supports weight management and overall health. The typical daily fluid intake guideline is about 13 cups for healthy men and 9 cups for healthy women. This principle does not apply to people with advanced CKD.

Principle 12: Engage in Regular Exercise

Regular exercise enhances insulin sensitivity and helps manage blood sugar levels. It also supports mental health and mood, increasing energy, reducing stress, and improving sleep.

Principle 13: Consume Nuts Regularly

Nuts are packed with essential nutrients, including mono- and polyunsaturated fats and protein, and are beneficial for managing type 2 diabetes and cardiovascular diseases.

Principle 14: Limit Red Meat and Ensure Adequate Protein

While red meat can be included in a balanced diet, it is advisable to moderate its consumption due to potential associations with chronic diseases. Opt for a variety of protein sources to ensure a balanced diet.

Principle 15: Exercise Caution with Alcohol Consumption

Manage alcohol intake carefully, as it can significantly disrupt blood sugar levels control and interact with diabetes medications. Understanding the effects of alcohol on glucose metabolism and its potential interactions with medications is vital for maintaining blood sugar control.

COMMON QUESTIONS & ANSWERS

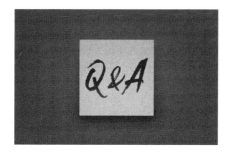

UNDERSTANDING GLYCEMIC INDEX AND GLYCEMIC LOAD

How can the Glycemic Index help in managing diabetes? The Glycemic Index (GI) helps manage diabetes by guiding individuals to choose foods that have a minimal impact on blood glucose levels. Low-GI diets are associated with lower glycated hemoglobin (HbA1c), indicating better blood glucose control and fewer hypoglycemia episodes. This approach can reduce medication needs, lower the risk of devastating complications, and enhance the quality of life for people with diabetes.

What factors influence the Glycemic Index of a food? The GI of food is influenced by the type of carbohydrate (simple vs. complex), processing methods, cooking techniques, and nutrient composition (e.g., fat and fiber). Whole grains typically have a lower GI than processed grains, and less processing or shorter cooking times usually result in a lower GI.

How does the ripeness of fruits and vegetables affect their GI and GL? Ripeness increases the sugar content of fruits and vegetables, raising their GI. Choosing less ripe options can lower the overall GI of the diet.

How can cooking methods alter the GI of foods? Cooking methods significantly affect the GI of foods. For example, boiling usually results in a lower GI than baking or frying. Cooking pasta 'al dente' (slightly firm) reduces its GI because the firmer texture slows digestion and glucose absorption.

How do food processing methods, such as milling and refining grains, impact the GI? Milling and refining grains remove bran and germ, reducing fiber content and increasing the GI. Whole grains digest and absorb more slowly due to their intact fiber, leading to more stable blood glucose levels.

How does the concept of 'al dente' cooking affect the GI of pasta? Cooking pasta 'al dente' reduces its GI because the firmer texture slows digestion and glucose absorption compared to fully cooked pasta, helping manage blood sugar levels more effectively.

What is the difference in GI between eating raw fruits and vegetables versus consuming them as juices? Eating raw fruits and vegetables generally results in a lower GI than consuming them as juices. Juicing removes fiber, which accelerates sugar digestion and absorption, causing more rapid blood glucose spikes. Whole fruits and vegetables retain fiber, leading to a slower increase in blood sugar levels.

Why do some foods have a high GI but a low-GL, and how should

they be incorporated into a diet? Foods with a high GI but low-GL contain relatively few carbohydrates per serving. These can be balanced with low-GI, higher-fiber foods in a diet to reduce the overall impact on blood sugar levels.

How does dehydration or drying fruits and vegetables affect their GL? Dehydrating or drying fruits and vegetables concentrates their sugars, potentially raising their GL compared to fresh versions. The effect varies based on the dehydration process and the specific fruit or vegetable.

How do sprouting grains or seeds before consuming them affect their GI? Sprouting grains or seeds alters their nutritional profile, reducing carbohydrate content and increasing fiber, which can lower the GI.

What are Advanced Glycation End-products (AGEs), and how do they relate to the GI of foods? Advanced Glycation End-products (AGEs) are compounds formed when proteins or fats interact with sugars. While not directly related to the GI of foods, high-AGE diets can worsen diabetes complications and inflammation. Cooking methods that use lower temperatures and more moisture, such as boiling or steaming, produce fewer AGEs than dry-heat methods like grilling or roasting.

What are the latest research findings on the low-GL diet and its impact on diabetes management? Recent research supports low-GL diets for diabetes management, highlighting improvements in glycemic control and insulin sensitivity. Such diets are linked to a reduced risk of type 2 diabetes complications, improved cholesterol levels, and overall health.

NUTRITIONAL STRATEGIES FOR BLOOD SUGAR MANAGEMENT

What are the benefits of following a low-GL diabetes diet for someone with diabetes? A low-GL diet provides several benefits for individuals with diabetes, such as improved glycemic control, reduced risk of hypoglycemic episodes, enhanced lipid profiles, and a lower likelihood of diabetes-related complications. Additionally, it aids in weight management, which is essential for overall diabetes care.

What strategies can be used to estimate the GI of a food if the value is not available in tables? To estimate the GI of foods not listed in tables, evaluate the food's fiber content, processing level, and cooking method. Generally, less processed foods, higher in fiber, and those cooked in ways that maintain their structure (e.g., boiling instead of frying) tend to have a lower GI.

How can meal timing and frequency impact blood sugar control? Meal timing and frequency play a crucial role in blood sugar control. Eating smaller, more regular meals can help stabilize blood glucose levels throughout the day, particularly when these meals consist of low-GL foods. This approach reduces the large blood sugar fluctuations often associated with larger, less frequent meals high in GL.

What is the impact of alcohol and caffeine on blood sugar levels? Caffeine can impair blood glucose management in individuals with type 2 diabetes, potentially raising serum insulin, proinsulin, and C-peptide levels. In contrast, moderate alcohol consumption generally does not adversely affect blood glucose control and may even lower fasting serum insulin levels in those with type 2 diabetes.

How can someone with diabetes effectively incorporate low-GL principles when dining out? When dining out, individuals with diabetes can follow low-GL principles by: a.) Choosing dishes with whole grains, legumes, or vegetables are primary ingredients. b.) Requesting dressings and sauces on the side to better control intake. c.) Preferring grilled, baked, or steamed dishes over fried options. d.)

Starting with a salad or vegetable-based soup to fill up on lower GL items.

What are the best low-GL snacks for managing hunger between meals? The best low-GL snacks for managing hunger include: a.) Nuts and seeds. b.) Greek yogurt c.) Fresh fruit. d.) Vegetables with hummus. e.) Whole grain homemade crackers with cheese or nut butter. These snacks deliver a consistent energy source and aid manage hunger between meals.

How can one balance a vegetarian or vegan diet with low-GL principles? Balancing a vegetarian or vegan diet with low-GL principles involves selecting plant-based foods that are naturally low in GL, such as whole grains, legumes, nuts, seeds, fruits, and vegetables. Incorporating these foods into your meal planning can assist in stabilizing blood sugar levels while following a vegetarian or vegan dietary regimen.

Can adding fats or oils to meals affect the GL, and in what way? Adding fats or oils to meals can reduce the GL by delaying carbohydrate absorption, thus moderating blood sugar spikes. It's important to select healthy fats and consider the overall calorie content of the meal to maintain a balanced diet.

Can the glycemic response to a meal be moderated by the order in which foods are eaten? The order of food consumption can influence the glycemic response. Eating proteins and vegetables before carbohydrates can result in a lower glycemic response than consuming carbohydrates first or all meal components together, offering a simple dietary modification to enhance glycemic control.

How do natural sweeteners (e.g., stevia, xylitol) compare to sugar in terms of GI? Natural sweeteners like stevia and xylitol have a lower GI than regular sugar. Stevia, a non-nutritive sweetener, has a GI of zero, making it an excellent option for blood sugar control. Xylitol, a sugar alcohol, offers a sweet taste with less impact on the glycemic response.

PART IV
DIETARY GUIDELINES AND MEAL PLANNING PRINCIPLES

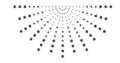

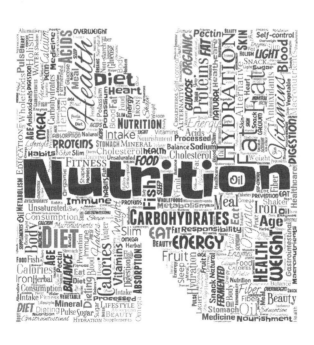

MEAL PLANNING GUIDELINES – THE THREE-TIERED APPROACH TO DIABETES MEAL PLANNING

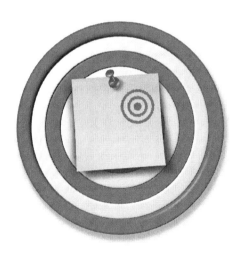

Effective Diabetes Meal Planning: A Comprehensive Guide to Managing Blood Sugar

Effective diabetes meal planning is crucial for maintaining stable blood sugar levels and driving positive health outcomes. This guide introduces a structured, two-phase approach to dietary management using glycemic index (GI), glycemic load (GL), and net carb values, enabling readers to progress from beginner to advanced strategies.

Overview of the Structured Approach:

- **Phase 1: Basic Level** - This initial phase provides straightforward tools such as diabetes-friendly food lists, each food with 15-20 grams carb equivalent serving sizes. It simplifies the introduction to a low-GL diet, focusing on easy-to-follow guidelines and basic food categorizations.
- **Phase 2: Advanced Level** - Building upon the basics, this phase offers a comprehensive glycemic index, glycemic load, and net carb counter. It expands the dietary toolkit, providing detailed nutritional data for a broader range of foods and helping readers fine-tune their meal planning based on more specific dietary needs.

PHASE 1: LOW-GL DIABETES FOOD LISTS

"Low-GL Diabetes Food Lists" offers an accessible starting point for those new to diabetes-conscious diets. It groups essential food categories—vegetables, fruits, grains, dairy, and proteins—into clear, easy-to-understand lists. Each food group is labeled either Low GI and Low-GL or Medium GI and Low-GL, indicating optimal choices for stable blood sugar levels. This section eschews complex jargon for straightforward, actionable information, making it a valuable resource for those overwhelmed by more detailed dietary planning. Foods are divided into five food groups: vegetables, Fruits, Grains, Dairy and Plant-based alternatives, and Protein Foods.

PHASE 2: COMPREHENSIVE TOOLS AND DETAILED GI, GL AND NET CARB DATA

The GI, GL, & Net Carb Counter in Phase 2 goes beyond basic lists, offering precise information on the glycemic impact of over 4,000 foods. This tool encourages moderation and informed choices, recommending that daily intake of foods with a GL over 20 be minimized, and aligns with CDC guidelines to limit added sugars. It also provides practical, patient-tested insights into selecting and consuming foods that support a low-GL diet, enhancing usability and adherence to healthy dietary practices.

This structured approach to meal planning equips you with the necessary knowledge, ressources and tools to effectively manage diabetes through diet. Each phase of meal planning builds progressively, ensuring a comprehensive integration of diabetes-friendly foods to align with your health goals.

15

DIETARY GUIDELINES AND THE STRUCTURED APPROACH OF THE LOW GL DIABETES DIET

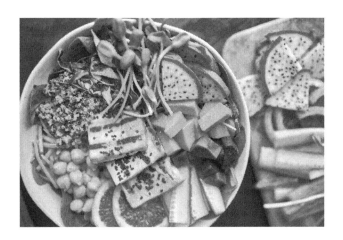

ALIGNMENT WITH CURRENT DIETARY GUIDELINES

The GL Diabetes Diet is fully aligned with the Dietary Guidelines for Americans 2020-2025, which advocate for a balanced diet that emphasizes a consistent intake of nutrient-dense foods from the five food groups while limiting added sugars, saturated fats, and sodium to promote healthy weight management. Although these guidelines do not address diabetes management directly, they provide foundational principles that are highly relevant and adaptable for a diabetes-friendly diet.

ADAPTATIONS TO COMPLEMENT THE LOW-GL DIABETES DIET:

- **Healthy Fats Over Saturated Fats:** For people with diabetes, who are at a higher risk of cardiovascular disease, it is crucial to replace saturated fats with healthy fats found in various foods.
- **Sodium and Blood Pressure Management:** Limiting sodium intake to under 2,300 milligrams daily is essential for individuals with diabetes to control blood pressure and lower the risk of cardiovascular disease.
- **Physical Activity:** Incorporating regular physical activity, as highlighted in the guidelines, is vital for managing diabetes. It enhances blood glucose control, lowers cardiovascular risk factors, and supports weight management.
- **Personalization to Individual Needs:** The guidelines underscore the importance of adapting dietary recommendations to personal preferences, cultural traditions, and specific health needs, allowing for tailoring food choices to dietary requirements and glycemic targets.
- **Focus on Whole Foods:** Emphasizing whole foods over processed options and supplements can aid in achieving a more nutrient-dense diet, which is beneficial for managing diabetes and enhancing overall health.

FOOD CATEGORIZATION

Aligned with the classification system from MyPlate.gov, foods are classified into five primary groups:

- Vegetables

- Fruits
- Grains
- Dairy and Plant-based Alternatives
- Protein Foods

A sixth category, 'Extras', has been introduced to encompass:

- Beverages
- Dressings and Oils
- Herbs and Spices

REFINING DIABETES MANAGEMENT WITH THE LOW-GL DIABETES DIETARY GUIDELINES

Building on adaptations and categorizations designed to support a comprehensive approach to diabetes management, the Low-GL Diabetes Dietary Guidelines introduce an effective meal planning strategy tailored for those managing diabetes. Key components include:

- **Assessment of Nutritional Needs:** Begin by assessing individual caloric needs based on age, sex, weight, activity level, and specific health goals to customize the diet plan and prevent excessive blood sugar fluctuations.
- **Adhering to the 15 Core Principles of the Low-GL Diabetes Diet:**
- Adopt principles that encompass everything from selecting the right types of foods to maintaining the proper balance of nutrients for optimal health and blood sugar management.
- **Balanced Meals Across Food Groups:** Organize meals with a balanced combination of carbs, proteins, and lipids to ensure nutritional completeness and maintain stable blood sugar levels throughout the day.
- **Scheduled Eating Times:** Establish regular meal and snack

times to prevent unexpected drops or spikes in blood glucose levels, enhancing metabolic control.

- **Strategic Snacking:** Schedule nutritious, well-timed snacks to control hunger and avoid overeating at main meals.
- **Hydration:** Adequate fluid intake is crucial for regulating blood sugar levels and preventing dehydration.
- **Monitoring and Adjustment:** Regularly monitor blood glucose levels to evaluate the effectiveness of the meal plan and make necessary dietary adjustments.
- **Educational Resources and Support:** Utilize resources like the Diabetes Food Hub endorsed by the American Diabetes Association (ADA) for diabetes-friendly recipes and meal planning ideas, and seek support from dietitians or diabetes educators for personalized advice.
- **Typical Serving Sizes** Detailed guidelines with typical serving sizes for each food group will be provided in upcoming chapters.

RECIPES

This book and none of my publications include a cookbook or specific recipes section. Instead, I guide patients and readers to online resources that are not only free but also reliable and effective. I particularly recommend the Diabetes Food Hub (https://www. diabetesfoodhub.org/), endorsed by the American Diabetes Association (ADA), as a valuable tool for finding diabetes-friendly recipes and meal planning ideas.

16

MACRONUTRIENT DISTRIBUTION FOR YOUR LOW GL DIABETES DIET

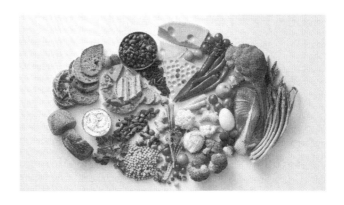

CALCULATING MACRONUTRIENT DISTRIBUTION FOR A LOW-GL DIABETES DIET

Follow these comprehensive instructions to calculate your macronutrient distribution for a low-GL diabetes diet. This guide will assist you through manual calculations and highlight how online tools can simplify the process.

92

STEP 1: MEASURE YOUR BASAL METABOLIC RATE (BMR)

Start by calculating your BMR, which reflects the amount of calories your body needs to fulfill basic life-sustaining functions like breathing, circulation, and cell production when at rest. Use the Mifflin-St Jeor equation for manual calculations.

For Men:

$$BMR = 10 \times \text{weight (kg)} + 6.25 \times \text{height (cm)} - 5 \times \text{age (y)} + 5$$

For Women:

$$BMR = 10 \times \text{weight (kg)} + 6.25 \times \text{height (cm)} - 5 \times \text{age (y)} - 161$$

Alternatively, you can use a reliable online BMR calculator like MyFitnessPal (https://www.myfitnesspal.com/tools/bmr-calculator), which computes these values for you upon entering your weight, height, age, and sex.

STEP 2: DETERMINE TOTAL DAILY ENERGY EXPENDITURE (TDEE)

Multiply your BMR by the relevant activity factor to calculate your TDEE. This measurement adjusts for your daily activity and exercise level, providing a more accurate estimate of your total caloric needs.

- Sedentary (little or no exercise): BMR × 1.2
- Lightly active (light exercise/sports 1-3 days/week): BMR × 1.375
- Moderately active (moderate exercise/sports 3-5 days/week): BMR × 1.55
- Very active (hard exercise/sports 6-7 days a week): BMR × 1.725
- Super active (very hard exercise/physical job & exercise 2x a day): BMR × 1.9

For convenience, use online TDEE calculators such as **TDEE Calculator** (https://tdeecalculator.net/), or **MyFitnessPal** (https://www.myfitnesspal.com/tools/bmr-calculator) to automatically factor in your activity level and provide an estimate.

STEP 3: CALCULATE MACRONUTRIENT DISTRIBUTION

With your TDEE calculated, allocate your calories among carbohydrates, proteins, and fats, prioritizing the quality of these macronutrients:

Carbohydrates: Aim for 45-50% of your total calories. Choose high-quality carbohydrates that have a low glycemic load.

Proteins: Your protein needs can vary:

- Normal weight without CKD: 0.8 to 1.2 grams per kg body weight.
- Overweight or obese: 1.5 to 2 grams per kg body weight.
- With early-stage CKD: 0.8 to 1 gram per kg body weight.
- Advanced CKD: 0.6 to 0.8 grams per kg body weight.

Fats: Allocate the remaining calories to fats, focusing on sources rich in monounsaturated and polyunsaturated fats.

STEP 4: CONVERT MACRONUTRIENT PERCENTAGES INTO GRAMS

To translate the calorie percentages into grams:

- Carbohydrates and proteins provide 4 calories per gram.
- Lipids or Fats provide 9 calories per gram.

For a 2000-calorie diet:

- **Carbohydrates:** 50% of 2000 calories = 1000 calories $\rightarrow \frac{1000 \text{ calories}}{4 \text{ cal/g}} =$ 250 grams
- **Proteins:** 20% of 2000 calories = 400 calories $\rightarrow \frac{400 \text{ calories}}{4 \text{ cal/g}} = 100$ grams
- **Fats:** 30% of 2000 calories = 600 calories $\rightarrow \frac{600 \text{ calories}}{9 \text{ cal/g}} = 67$ grams

STEP 5: CONTINUOUSLY MONITOR AND ADJUST

Regularly monitor your health and adjust your macronutrient intake as needed. This helps manage your diabetes effectively and aligns with your health goals. Pay particular attention to how your body responds to different macronutrient distributions and adjust based on your metabolic health, blood sugar responses, and overall well-being.

By following these detailed steps, you can tailor your diet to manage diabetes through a controlled and informed approach to macronutrient distribution. Whether you calculate manually or use online tools, consistency and regular adjustment based on real-world outcomes are key.

THE PLATE METHOD

THE IMPORTANCE OF PORTION CONTROL IN MANAGING DIABETES

Understanding portion control is essential for managing a diabetes diet, especially concerning the Glycemic Load (GL) of foods. It's important to recognize that even low-GL foods can cause significant glycemic responses if consumed in amounts larger than standard serving sizes. GL values are influenced by portion size; eating more than the typical serving can increase the meal's GL, raising glucose levels in the bloodstream.

For example, doubling the portion of a low-GL food item could escalate its glycemic impact to a medium or high level. This demonstrates that the glycemic impact of a food can substantially change with portion size, making adherence to recommended serving sizes crucial for maintaining stable blood sugar levels.

THE PLATE METHOD: SIMPLIFYING DIETARY MANAGEMENT

After exploring advanced techniques like calculating macronutrient distribution in the previous chapter, we introduce a simpler method for beginners to manage their diet effectively: the Plate Method.

The Plate Method Explained The Plate Method is a visually intuitive strategy for assembling balanced meals:

Vegetables: Half of your plate should consist of colorful, non-starchy vegetables such as leafy greens, peppers, and broccoli. These are nutrient-rich, fiber-dense, and low in calories and carbohydrates.

Protein: One-quarter of your plate should consist of lean protein sources (e.g., chicken, fish, tofu, or beans), which are crucial for tissue repair and help maintain muscle mass.

Carbohydrates: The remaining quarter should include carbohydrate-rich foods like whole grains (brown rice, quinoa) or starchy vegetables (sweet potatoes). These should be consumed in moderation to provide necessary energy without excessive glucose spikes.

ADVANTAGES AND LIMITATIONS OF THE PLATE METHOD

This method offers a straightforward approach to healthy eating, promoting balanced macronutrient intake and aiding in weight and glycemic control. However, it may not provide the detailed guidance needed for individuals with specific health conditions like chronic kidney disease, or those who require strict blood sugar management. Despite this, the Plate Method remains an effective and appealing strategy for those new to dietary management, offering a strong foundation for initiating a low-GL diabetes diet.

18

CRAFTING A ONE-DAY MEAL PLAN

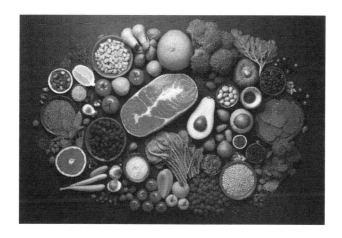

This chapter offers a step-by-step tutorial on developing daily or weekly meal plans that align with the principles of the low-GL diabetes diet. Rather than supplying rigid 7-day or 4-week meal plans, it empowers you to design customized meal plans that consider your preferences, budget constraints, seasonal food availability, and specific health conditions, such as food intolerances.

DETAILED ONE-DAY MEAL PLAN: BALANCING NUTRITION AND FLEXIBILITY

Objective: Enable effective diabetes management through personalized diet planning. This plan is not just about adhering to dietary restrictions but about integrating healthy choices seamlessly into your lifestyle, enhancing both glycemic control and overall well-being.

Key Benefits:

- **Carbohydrate Management:** Aims for 45-50% of daily calories from carbohydrates, ensuring stable blood sugar levels.
- **Protein Intake:** Ensures adequate daily protein intake for tissue repair and muscle maintenance.
- **Healthy Fats:** Focuses on fats that support cardiovascular health and provide long-lasting energy.

Plan Compliance Features:

Low-GL Foods: Incorporates primarily low-GL ingredients to minimize blood sugar spikes.

Safe Cooking Methods: Emphasizes cooking methods that maintain nutrient integrity and avoid creating harmful compounds.

Core Principles Adherence: Complies with established dietary guidelines to enhance the effectiveness of the diet.

Meal Breakdown for a 2000-Calorie Diet:

Total Daily Carbohydrates: Approximately 225 grams, ensuring about 45% of daily caloric intake, and including 20 to 35 grams of fiber to optimize digestive health and glycemic response.

BELOW IS THE MEAL PLAN:

Total Daily Carbohydrates: Approximately 225 grams, including 20 to 35 grams of fiber. 225 grams equates to 900 calories because each gram is 4 calories. On a 2000-calorie diet, this ensures that 45% of daily calories come from carbohydrates.

Breakfast:

- **Dish:** Oatmeal with Berries, Almonds, and Chia Seeds
- **Serving Size:** ¾ cup cooked oatmeal, 1 cup fresh berries, 10 almonds, 1 tablespoon chia seeds
- **Carbohydrates:** Approx. 50 grams
- **Description:** Oats provide a slow-releasing carbohydrate source. Berries add fiber, almonds contribute healthy fats and protein, and chia seeds increase the fiber content, making for a nutrient-dense start to the day.

Morning Snack:

- **Dish:** Greek Yogurt with Raspberries and a Drizzle of Honey
- **Serving Size:** 1 cup Greek yogurt, 1 cup raspberries, 1 teaspoon honey
- **Carbohydrates:** Approx. 30 grams
- **Description:** Greek yogurt is high in protein, raspberries are rich in fiber, and a small amount of honey provides a natural sweetener without significantly impacting the glycemic load.

Lunch:

- **Dish:** Quinoa Salad with Mixed Greens, Cherry Tomatoes, Grilled Chicken, Avocado, and Vinaigrette
- **Serving Size:** 1 cup cooked quinoa, 2 cups mixed greens, ½ cup cherry tomatoes, 4 oz grilled chicken, ½ sliced avocado, 2 tablespoons vinaigrette

- **Carbohydrates:** Approx. 50 grams
- **Description:** Quinoa and mixed greens serve as low GI carbohydrate sources, chicken provides protein, avocado offers healthy fats, and tomatoes add additional fiber and nutrients.

Afternoon Snack:

- **Dish:** Whole Wheat Pita with Hummus and Sliced Cucumber
- **Serving Size:** 1 small whole wheat pita, 3 tablespoons hummus, ½ cup sliced cucumber
- **Carbohydrates:** Approx. 30 grams
- **Description:** Whole wheat pita provides complex carbohydrates and fiber, hummus contributes protein and fat, and cucumber offers hydration and additional nutrients.

Dinner:

- **Dish:** Grilled Salmon with Sweet Potato and Steamed Broccoli
- **Serving Size:** 5 oz grilled salmon, 1 medium sweet potato, 1 cup steamed broccoli
- **Carbohydrates:** Approx. 45 grams
- **Description:** Salmon is rich in omega-3 fatty acids, sweet potato is a high-fiber carbohydrate source, and broccoli is packed with nutrients and fiber for a balanced meal.

Evening Snack:

- **Dish:** Pear with a Slice of Cheese
- **Serving Size:** 1 medium pear, 1 slice of cheese
- **Carbohydrates:** Approx. 20 grams
- **Description:** Pear provides a low GI, fiber-rich fruit option, paired with cheese for protein and fat, rounding out the day with a balanced snack.

STEP-BY-STEP GUIDE TO DESIGNING DIABETES-FRIENDLY MEAL PLANS

This section details a structured approach to meal planning that caters to varying stages of dietary management and personalizes the diet to your unique nutritional needs and management goals.

STEP 1: FOOD SELECTION

Start with the diabetes-friendly food lists or use the detailed GI, GL, and net carb data, which offers detailed information about serving size, GI and GL values, and net carb content.

STEP 2: CALORIC NEEDS DETERMINATION

Use online tools like TDEE Calculator or MyFitnessPal to calculate your daily caloric requirements, helping tailor your meal plan to your health needs and lifestyle.

STEP 3: MACRONUTRIENT DISTRIBUTION PLANNING

Allocate 45-50% of your daily calories to carbohydrates, using the Plate Method as a visual aid to ensure a balanced intake of macros.

STEP 4: SERVING SIZE COMPLIANCE

Follow recommended serving sizes to achieve the desired balance of nutrients and maintain glycemic control.

STEP 5: CORE PRINCIPLES CHECKLIST

Develop a checklist based on the 15 core principles, and use it to ensure each meal aligns with these guidelines for comprehensive diabetes management.

15 core principles Checklist

STEP	TASK	DONE
01	Check for Low-Glycemic Index Foods in each meal	☐
02	Increase Olive Oil Consumption in your cooking.	☐
03	Limit Added Sugar Intake throughout the day.	☐
04	Reduce Sodium Intake by choosing low-salt options.	☐
05	Include Polyphenol-Rich Foods in your diet.	☐
06	Select Flavonoid-Rich Foods when choosing fruits and vegetables.	☐
07	Use Healthy Fats in meal preparations.	☐
08	Ensure Omega-3 Fatty Acids are present in your meals.	☐
09	Add Anti-inflammatory Spices to enhance flavors naturally.	☐
10	Avoid Foods with Artificial Trans Fats entirely	☐
11	Drink plenty of water to maintain hydration.	☐
12	Plan for Regular Physical Activity each day.	☐
13	Incorporate Regular Nut Consumption into snacks or meals.	☐
14	Control Red Meat Intake but ensure adequate protein	☐
15	Monitor Alcohol Consumption, keeping it minimal and occasional.	☐

Step 6: Cooking Methods and Times

Select cooking methods that do not increase the glycemic index, such as steaming and boiling. Monitor cooking times to avoid overcooking, which can affect the GI of foods.

IMPLEMENTATION TIPS:

Plan Ahead: Dedicate weekly time slots to meal planning to ensure consistency.

Batch Cooking: Prepare meals in batches to save time and maintain consistency in nutrition and taste.

Regular Reviews: Continually assess your meal plan's effectiveness and make adjustments based on health outcomes and consultations with healthcare providers.

By methodically applying these steps, you can create personalized, effective meal plans that not only help manage your diabetes but also integrate healthily into your lifestyle, promoting long-term well-being and stability in blood sugar levels.

PART V
LOW GL DIABETES DIET
FOOD LISTS

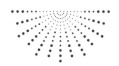

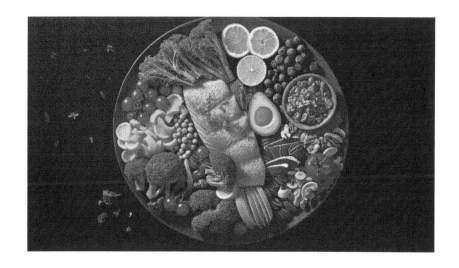

19

THE VEGETABLES DIABETES-FRIENDLY FOOD LISTS

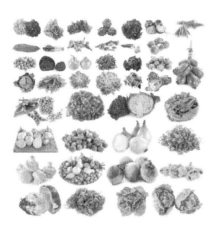

The low-GL diabetes diet places strong emphasis on the regular and varied consumption of vegetables, due to their nutrient-rich composition. Vegetables are particularly notable for their high concentration of dietary fiber, vitamins, minerals and a range of beneficial phytochemicals, including polyphenols, flavonoids, beta-carotene, anthocyanidins and carotenoids. Research by Darmon et al (2005) highlights that fruits and vegetables achieve high nutrient density scores mainly because they are rich in nutrients relative to their low energy content. They also have a favorable nutrient/price ratio, providing vital nutrients at a reasonable cost compared to other food groups.

According to MyPlate.gov, vegetables are classified into five subgroups, each defined by their specific nutrient contributions:

1. **Dark green vegetables:** These foods are packed with essential vitamins (A, C, E, and K) and minerals (iron, calcium, magnesium, and potassium). Their potent antioxidant properties help prevent chronic diseases, including various cancers and heart disease.
2. **Red and orange vegetables:** Rich in vitamins A and C, these vegetables are renowned for their powerful antioxidant properties, which help prevent disease.
3. **Pulses (beans, peas, lentils):** Excellent sources of plant-based protein and fiber, legumes have a low glycemic index, which promotes stable blood sugar management and makes them essential for diabetics.
4. **Starchy vegetables:** Although these vegetables are higher in carbohydrates, they remain a crucial part of a balanced diet, providing essential nutrients. For people with diabetes, careful portion control is essential.
5. **Other vegetables:** This category includes a variety of vegetables, each with a unique nutritional profile. They are generally less carbohydrate-rich than their starchy counterparts, and rich in vitamins and minerals.

STARCHY VS. NON-STARCHY VEGETABLES IN A LOW-GL DIABETES DIET

The key distinction between starchy and non-starchy vegetables within a low-GL diabetes diet centers around their carbohydrate content, effects on blood sugar levels, and implications for weight management. Starchy vegetables, such as potatoes, corn, peas, plantains, yams, carrots, sweet potatoes, and parsnips, are higher in carbohydrates and calories. While the starch in these vegetables—a complex carbohydrate—is converted into glucose by the body, it is their overall higher carbohydrate content that typically results in a greater glycemic load (GL). Thus, careful portion control of starchy vegetables is crucial in a low-GL diet.

NUTRITIONAL PROFILES:

Starchy Vegetables:

- **Calories:** Higher calorie content due to more carbohydrates.
- **Carbohydrates:** Contains complex carbs which provide sustained energy.
- **Fiber:** Often rich in fiber, particularly in their skins.
- **Nutrients:** High in vitamin C, potassium, and vitamin B6.
- **Energy Density:** Higher carbohydrate content leads to more energy per unit weight, thus a higher GL.

Non-Starchy Vegetables:

- **Calories:** Lower in calories and carbohydrates.
- **Carbohydrates:** Contain less starch and more fiber, impacting blood sugar minimally.
- **Fiber:** High fiber content supports digestion and satiety.
- **Nutrients:** Non-starchy vegetables are packed with vitamins (A, C, K, and folate) and minerals (iron, calcium, potassium, and magnesium).
- **Energy Density:** Less dense in calories and carbohydrates, beneficial for weight management.

Density Differences:

Starchy Vegetables: Offer a heartier, denser texture, providing more satisfying meals.

Non-Starchy Vegetables: Typically more water-rich, leading to a lighter texture, ideal for calorie control and weight management.

HEALTH IMPLICATIONS:

Incorporating non-starchy vegetables is especially beneficial for managing type 2 diabetes mellitus (T2DM), as supported by the twin cycle hypothesis, which suggests that weight loss is key to reversing insulin resistance and beta-cell dysfunction seen in T2DM. Non-starchy vegetables, with their lower GL and calorie content, are pivotal in dietary strategies focused on weight loss and optimal blood sugar management. Aligning with the low-GL diet principles, these vegetables minimize glycemic variability, enhancing diabetes management and promoting long-term health.

Extensive research confirms that a diet rich in fruits and vegetables not only benefits overall health but also reduces the risk of developing complications related to type 2 diabetes. The protective effects of these foods are largely attributed to their antioxidants, fiber, and nutrient density.

BEANS, PEAS, AND LENTILS IN THE LOW-GL DIABETES DIET

Beans, peas, and lentils are invaluable for those following a low-GL diabetes diet due to their beneficial nutritional properties.

Benefits of Including Beans, Peas, and Lentils:

- **Low Glycemic Index:** These legumes typically have a low GI, which means they cause a slower and less pronounced rise in blood sugar levels post-meal.

- **High Fiber Content:** The abundant fiber helps slow-GLucose absorption, improving overall digestive health and prolonging satiety.
- **Rich in Protein:** Essential for blood sugar management, protein helps enhance satiety and prevents spikes in blood sugar levels after meals.
- **Nutrient Density:** Beans, peas, and lentils are packed with essential nutrients, including iron, potassium, magnesium, and B vitamins, supporting overall health and not just diabetes management.

PORTION SIZES AND INTAKE RECOMMENDATIONS

Proper understanding of portion sizes is crucial for maintaining stable blood sugar levels, particularly in relation to carbohydrate content in meals. Ideally, each serving of these legumes should contain no more than 15 grams of carbohydrates. It is concerning that many people do not meet the recommended daily intake of vegetables and legumes, which can significantly affect overall health and diabetes management.

GUIDELINES FOR VEGETABLE AND LEGUME INTAKE FOR DIABETES MANAGEMENT:

Carbohydrate Management: Each serving is recommended to contain approximately 15 grams of carbohydrates to align with dietary guidelines for diabetes management.

Daily Recommendations: Generally, adults should aim to consume at least 2-3 cups of vegetables and legumes each day as part of a balanced diet to ensure adequate nutrient intake and to aid in blood sugar regulation.

Here's a table summarizing the serving sizes for different vegetable subgroups, each designed to contain no more than 15 grams of carbohydrates and the general daily recommendation:

Vegetable Subgroup	Serving Size	Carbohydrate Content (Approx.)	Daily Recommended Servings
Dark-Green Vegetables	1 cup (cooked or raw)	<5 grams	1-2 servings
Red and Orange Vegetables	1/2 cup (cooked)	15 grams	1-2 servings
Starchy Vegetables	1/2 cup (cooked)	15 grams	1 serving
Beans and Peas (Legumes)	1/3 cup (cooked)	15 grams	1 serving
Other Vegetables	1 cup (raw or cooked)	<5 grams	1-2 servings

THE LOW-GL DIABETES FOOD LISTS

Dark-Green Vegetables

- **Amaranth Leaves (all forms)** — Low GI, low-GL. Rich in vitamins A, C, folate, and dietary fiber.
- **Arugula (Rocket) (all forms)** — Low GI, negligible GL. High in calcium, potassium, folate, and vitamin K.
- **Asparagus (all forms)** — Low GI, low-GL. High in vitamin A, C, E, and K, and folate and fiber.
- **Beet Greens (all forms)** — Low GI, low-GL. High in fiber, vitamin A, vitamin C, and potassium.
- **Bok Choy (Chinese Chard) (all forms)** — Low GI, very low-GL. High in vitamins A, C, K, calcium and iron.
- **Broccoli (all forms)** — Low GI, very low-GL. High in vitamin C, vitamin K, fiber and potassium.
- **Brussels Sprouts (all forms)** — Low GI, low-GL. High in fiber, vitamins C and K, and numerous nutrients.

- **Chamnamul (all forms)** — Low GI, low-GL. Typically high in vitamins and minerals.
- **Chard (all forms)** — Low GI, low-GL. Great source of vitamins A, C, and K, magnesium, manganese, iron, and dietary fiber.
- **Collards (all forms)** — Low GI, low-GL. High in vitamin A, C, and K, and fiber.
- **Dandelion Greens (all forms)** — Low GI, low-GL. Packed with calcium, iron, fiber, and vitamins A and K.
- **Endive (all forms)** — Low GI, very low-GL. High in fiber and vitamins A and K.
- **Kale (all forms)** — Low GI, low-GL. Very high in vitamins A, C, K, and significant amounts of minerals and antioxidants.
- **Kohlrabi Greens (all forms)** — Low GI, low-GL. Contains fiber, vitamins A, C, and K.
- **Mesclun Greens (typically raw)** — Low GI, negligible GL. A mix that usually includes a variety of nutrient-rich, low GI leafy greens.
- **Mustard Greens (all forms)** — Low GI, low-GL. High in vitamin A, C, and K, fiber, and antioxidants.
- **Nasturtium Leaves (typically raw)** — Low GI, negligible GL. Known for their high vitamin C content and unique peppery flavor.
- **Poke Greens (all forms)** — Low GI, low-GL. Must be cooked properly to neutralize toxins; high in vitamins A and C once safely prepared.
- **Rapini (Broccoli Raab) (all forms)** — Low GI, low-GL. High in vitamins A, C, and K, and includes beneficial plant compounds.
- **Romaine Lettuce (all forms)** — Very low GI, negligible GL. High in fiber, vitamins A, C, K, and folate.
- **Sorrel (all forms)** — Low GI, low-GL. Rich in vitamin A, C and dietary fiber.
- **Spinach (all forms)** — Low GI, low-GL. Extremely high in vitamin K, and high in manganese, folate, and iron.

- **Swiss Chard (all forms)** — Low GI, low-GL. High in vitamin A, C, and K, magnesium, potassium and fiber.
- **Taro Leaves (all forms)** — Low GI, low-GL when cooked. High in vitamin A, C, fiber, and several other essential nutrients.
- **Turnip Greens (all forms)** — Low GI, low-GL. High in vitamin A, C, K, calcium, folate, and fiber.
- **Watercress (all forms)** — Very low GI, negligible GL. High in vitamins A, C, and K.

Red and Orange Vegetables

- **Acorn Squash (all forms)** — Moderate GI, low-GL when consumed in small portions. High in vitamin A, C, and dietary fiber.
- **Beets (all forms)** — Medium GI, low to moderate GL. High in fiber, folate, and manganese, making them beneficial for blood sugar control when eaten in moderation.
- **Butternut Squash (all forms)** — Moderate GI, low-GL in controlled portions. High in vitamins A, C and fiber.
- **Calabaza (all forms)** — Moderate GI, low-GL when portion-controlled. High in vitamin A, C, and fiber.
- **Carrots (all forms)** — Low to moderate GI, very low-GL. High in beta-carotene and fiber.
- **Chili Peppers (all forms)** — Low GI, negligible GL. High in vitamin C and B6, capsaicin, and antioxidants.
- **Hubbard Squash (all forms)** — Moderate GI, low-GL in controlled portions. High vitamin C and dietary fiber.
- **Orange Bell Peppers (all forms)** — Low GI, very low-GL. High in vitamin A, C, and fiber.
- **Orange Cauliflower (all forms)** — Low GI, very low-GL. Offers slightly higher beta-carotene than white varieties, along with high vitamin C and fiber content.

- **Paprika (from dried red peppers)** — Low GI, minimal GL. High in vitamin A, E, and capsaicin.
- **Peppadew Peppers (all forms)** — Moderate GI, low-GL. High in vitamin C and dietary fiber.
- **Persimmons (typically raw)** — Moderate GI, moderate GL. High in vitamin A and C and fiber.
- **Pumpkin (all forms)** — Low GI, low-GL. High in fiber and beta-carotene.
- **Radishes (typically raw)** — Very low GI, negligible GL. High in vitamin C and other minerals, with very low carbohydrate content, making them an excellent choice for snacks.
- **Red and Orange Bell Peppers (all forms)** — Low GI, very low-GL. High in vitamins A and C and fiber.
- **Red Bell Peppers (all forms)** — Low GI, very low-GL. Exceptionally high in vitamin C, with good amounts of fiber, and antioxidants.
- **Red Cabbage (all forms)** — Low GI, very low-GL. High in vitamin C, K, fiber, and anthocyanins.
- **Red Kuri Squash (all forms)** — Moderate GI, low-GL in small servings. High in beta-carotene, vitamins C, E, and fiber.
- **Red Onions (all forms)** — Low GI, low-GL. Contains quercetin and fiber.
- **Rutabaga (all forms)** — Low GI, low-GL. Nutrient-rich with potassium, fiber, and vitamin C.
- **Sweet Potatoes (all forms)** — Moderate GI, moderate GL depending on cooking method. High in vitamins A, C and fiber.
- **Tomatoes (all forms)** — Low GI, low-GL. High in lycopene, vitamin C, and potassium.
- **Winter Squash (all forms)** — Moderate GI, low-GL when consumed in controlled portions. High in vitamin A, C, fiber, and antioxidants..

Beans, Peas, Lentils

- **Beans (All Cooked from Dry)**: Beans are a diverse group that offers low-GL options with high fiber and protein content.
- **Peas (All Cooked from Dry)**: Like beans, peas are good source of protein and fiber.
- **Chickpeas (Garbanzo Beans) (All Cooked from Dry)**: High in both fiber and protein, chickpeas can help manage blood sugar levels effectively.
- **Lentils (All Cooked from Dry)**: Lentils are especially beneficial in a diabetes diet as they have one of the lowest glycemic indices among legumes and are rich in fiber and protein.
- **Black Beans (All Cooked from Dry)**: Known for their deep color and rich flavor, black beans also offer antioxidant benefits alongside fiber and protein.
- **Black-Eyed Peas (All Cooked from Dry)**: These beans are particularly high in potassium and fiber, aiding in cardiovascular and glycemic health.
- **Bayo Beans (All Cooked from Dry)**: A lesser-known variety, Bayo beans are nutritious and have similar benefits to more common beans, including stabilizing blood glucose levels.
- **Cannellini Beans (All Cooked from Dry)**: These white kidney beans are excellent for blood sugar control due to their high fiber content and protein.
- **Great Northern Beans (All Cooked from Dry)**: Another bean variety that is effective at managing blood sugar due to its low GI and high fiber.
- **Edamame (All Cooked from Dry)**: Young soybeans that are a great source of protein and fiber, making them ideal for diabetes management.
- **Kidney Beans (All Cooked from Dry)**: Rich in various nutrients including magnesium and potassium, kidney beans are effective in a low-GL diet.
- **Lima Beans (All Cooked from Dry)**: Known for their buttery

texture, lima beans are a good source of fiber and slow-digesting carbohydrates.

- **Mung Beans (All Cooked from Dry)**: These small green beans are packed with essential nutrients.
- **Pigeon Peas (All Cooked from Dry)**: Common in tropical regions, pigeon peas are used in many traditional dishes and support glycemic control with their high fiber and protein content.
- **Pinto Beans (All Cooked from Dry)**: Popular in Mexican cuisine, pinto beans are versatile and beneficial for blood sugar regulation.
- **Split Peas (All Cooked from Dry)**: A staple in soup, split peas are highly nutritious, offering both fiber and protein to maintain stable blood glucose levels.

Starchy Vegetables

- **Breadfruit (All Fresh or Frozen)**: Rich in carbohydrates and fiber, breadfruit can be a part of a balanced diabetes diet when portion control is practiced.
- **Burdock Root (All Fresh or Frozen)**: Known for its earthy flavor, it's low in calories and high in fiber.
- **Cassava (All Fresh or Frozen)**: Also known as yuca, cassava is high in carbohydrates and should be consumed in moderation. It offers a gluten-free starch alternative but is low in protein and other nutrients.
- **Jicama (All Fresh or Frozen)**: Low in calories and high in fiber, jicama can be a crunchy, satisfying addition to a diabetes-friendly diet.
- **Lotus Root (All Fresh or Frozen)**: Provides a modest amount of fiber and is a good source of vitamin C and potassium. Its unique texture makes it versatile in cooking.
- **Plantains (All Fresh or Frozen)**: Similar to bananas but

higher in starch, plantains must be cooked before eating and are best consumed in controlled portions to manage their impact on blood sugar.

- **Salsify (All Fresh or Frozen)**: Often referred to as the oyster plant due to its flavor, salsify is high in fiber and can be beneficial for blood sugar control.
- **Taro Root (Dasheen or Yautia) (All Fresh or Frozen)**: Rich in fiber and other nutrients, taro root has a lower glycemic index than many other starchy vegetables, making it suitable for a diabetes diet when used in moderation.
- **Water Chestnuts (All Fresh or Frozen)**: Though they are higher in carbohydrates, their crunchy texture and high water content make them less calorie-dense and can be included in small amounts in a diabetes-friendly diet.
- **Yam (All Fresh or Frozen)**: Yams are a good source of fiber and antioxidants, although they are higher in carbohydrates. They should be eaten in moderation within a diabetes diet.
- **Yucca (All Fresh or Frozen)**: Similar to cassava, yucca provides a high-energy carbohydrate source but lacks significant amounts of protein or fat, making it important to balance it with other nutrients.

1.6 Other Vegetables

- **Asparagus** (all fresh, frozen, cooked, or raw)
- **Avocado** (all fresh, frozen, cooked, or raw)
- **Bamboo shoots** (all fresh, frozen, cooked, or raw)
- **Beets** (all fresh, frozen, cooked, or raw)
- **Bitter melon** (all fresh, frozen, cooked, or raw)
- **Brussels sprouts** (all fresh, frozen, cooked, or raw)
- **Green cabbage** (all fresh, frozen, cooked, or raw)
- **Savoy cabbage** (all fresh, frozen, cooked, or raw)
- **Red cabbage** (all fresh, frozen, cooked, or raw)

- **Cactus pads** (all fresh, frozen, cooked, or raw)
- **Cauliflower** (all fresh, frozen, cooked, or raw)
- **Celery** (all fresh, frozen, cooked, or raw)
- **Chayote (mirliton)** (all fresh, frozen, cooked, or raw)
- **Cucumber** (all fresh, frozen, cooked, or raw)
- **Eggplant** (all fresh, frozen, cooked, or raw)
- **Green beans** (all fresh, frozen, cooked, or raw)
- **Kohlrabi** (all fresh, frozen, cooked, or raw)
- **Luffa** (all fresh, frozen, cooked, or raw)
- **Mushrooms** (all fresh, frozen, cooked, or raw)
- **Okra** (all fresh, frozen, cooked, or raw)
- **Onions** (all fresh, frozen, cooked, or raw)
- **Radish** (all fresh, frozen, cooked, or raw)
- **Rutabaga** (all fresh, frozen, cooked, or raw)
- **Seaweed** (all fresh, frozen, cooked, or raw)
- **Snow peas** (all fresh, frozen, cooked, or raw)
- **Summer squash** (all fresh, frozen, cooked, or raw)
- **Tomatillos** (all fresh, frozen, cooked, or raw)

THE FRUITS DIABETES-FRIENDLY FOOD LISTS

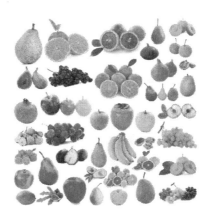

THE FRUIT FOOD GROUP AND THE LOW-GL DIABETES DIET

In accordance with MyPlate.gov, the fruit group encompasses all types of fruits, including whole fruits—fresh, frozen, or dried—canned fruits, and 100% fruit juices. For those on a low glycemic Load diabetes diet, emphasis is placed on whole fruits, which should make up at least 85% of daily fruit intake, rather than juices or processed fruit products. Whole fruits are preferred because they generally have lower GL values and a richer nutrient profile, both crucial for effective diabetes management.

Nutrient Density and Benefits of Whole Fruits

Whole fruits are packed with essential nutrients yet contain relatively few calories. They are excellent sources of vitamins and minerals such as vitamin C, potassium, and folate, and provide phytochemicals like phenols and antioxidants. These compounds play a key role in reducing oxidative stress and inflammation, which are vital for managing chronic conditions such as diabetes.

- **Phenolic Compounds:** Antioxidants in fruits that protect cells from oxidative damage.
- **Fiber Content:** Abundant in whole fruits, fiber slows sugar absorption and reduces the glycemic response.
- **Caloric Impact:** Whole fruits typically have fewer calories than processed fruit products, aiding in weight management, a key component of diabetes care.

Fruit Juice and Smoothies While 100% fruit juice is classified as part of the fruit group, it's recommended to limit its consumption in a low-GL diabetes diet due to its higher GL and absence of fiber, which is crucial for moderating glucose absorption. Smoothies, on the other hand, can be included in a nutritious diabetes diet when made with whole fruits, vegetables, and other low-GL ingredients. Incorporating protein and healthy fats into smoothies can help achieve a balanced macronutrient profile, stabilizing blood glucose levels.

Citrus Additions and Fruit Cocktails Integrating citrus fruits into juices or smoothies can reduce their GL, thanks to the vitamin C and flavonoids they contain, which provide metabolic and antioxidant benefits. The GL of fruit cocktails will depend on the types of fruits used and their preparation method. Opting for fresh fruit salads or those prepared with water rather than syrup is recommended to minimize the glycemic impact.

PORTION SIZES AND INTAKE RECOMMENDATIONS

Managing fruit intake is essential for people with diabetes due to the natural sugars in fruits, which can influence blood sugar levels. Adhering to appropriate serving sizes is crucial to ensure that each serving contains no more than 15 grams of carbohydrates, supporting diabetes management objectives.

Guidelines for Fruit Intake for Diabetes Management:

Carbohydrate Management: Each fruit serving is carefully portioned to provide about 15 grams of carbohydrates to aid in blood sugar control.

Daily Recommendations: Adults should aim to consume at least 1.5 to 2 cups of low-GL fruits daily as part of a balanced diet, aligning with diabetes management and overall health goals.

Here's a table summarizing the serving sizes for fruits, each designed to contain no more than 15 grams of carbohydrates, alongside the general daily recommendation:

Fruit Type	Serving Size	Carbohydrate Content (Approx.)	Daily Recommended Servings
Whole Fruit (small)	1 piece (e.g., an apple, orange)	15 grams	2 servings
Berries or Melons	1 cup (raw)	15 grams	2 servings
Dried Fruit	2 tablespoons	15 grams	1 serving
100% Fruit Juice	1/2 cup	15 grams	1 serving

For fruits that are naturally larger in size or have a higher water content, such as mango, papaya, watermelon, and melon, the serving sizes should indeed be adjusted to align with the low-GL diabetes diet. Since these fruits do not share a uniform nutritional profile, tailoring the serving sizes is essential to achieve the desired carbohydrate content.

Fruit Type	Serving Size	Total Carbohydrate Content	Fiber Content	Net Carbohydrate Content	Approximate Serving for 15g of Carbohydrates
Mango	1 cup (sliced, 165g)	28 grams	3 grams	25 grams	About 1/2 cup (82.5g)
Watermelon	1 cup (diced, 152g)	11.5 grams	0.5 grams	11 grams	Slightly more than 1 cup (165g)
Papaya	1 cup (cubed, 140g)	16 grams	2.5 grams	13.5 grams	Close to 1 cup (140g)
Melon (Cantaloupe)	1 cup (cubed, 160g)	13 grams	1.4 grams	11.6 grams	Slightly more than 1 cup (170g)
Honeydew Melon	1 cup (cubed, 170g)	15 grams	1.3 grams	13.7 grams	1 cup (170g)

Adjusting Fruit Portions for Low-GL Diabetes Diet

Mango, which is relatively high in carbohydrates, should be consumed in smaller portions compared to watermelon, which has fewer carbohydrates per cup and allows for a larger portion size. This approach helps maintain each serving at approximately 15 grams of carbohydrates. Similarly, with careful portioning, fruits like papaya, cantaloupe, and honeydew melon can be included in amounts close to 1 cup, aligning with the same carbohydrate target. Proper portion sizes for these fruits are crucial to fitting them within the low-GL diabetes framework, underscoring the importance of portion control.

Key Points:

Whole Fruits: Choosing whole fruits, especially those with skins, provides extra fiber which helps manage blood sugar levels by slowing the absorption of sugars.

Berries and Melons: These fruits are generally lower in carbohydrates per volume, allowing for larger portions that enhance satiety without significantly affecting blood sugar.

Dried Fruits and Juices: These options have a concentrated sugar content and should be consumed in smaller quantities. Always check labels for added sugars and opt for unsweetened varieties.

National Intake Recommendations:

Underconsumption Issue: Many Americans do not meet the recommended daily fruit intake, resulting in a deficit of essential nutrients and antioxidants. These components are crucial for reducing the risk of chronic diseases and enhancing overall health.

Monitoring fruit consumption carefully, choosing appropriate portions and types, is essential. Increasing fruit intake not only aids in diabetes management through controlled portions but also enhances overall health by supplying necessary vitamins, minerals, and dietary fiber. Achieving recommended daily servings of fruits can lead to a more balanced diet and improved health outcomes.

The Low-GL Diabetes Diet List

- **Apples (all fresh, frozen, dried fruits or 100% fruit juices)** — Low GI, good fiber content, carb content: low. Apples are rich in fiber, vitamin E, C, and antioxidants, which are crucial for oxidative stress reduction and immune support. Best consumed with the skin on for maximum fiber benefit.
- **Acai (all fresh, frozen, dried fruits or 100% fruit juices)** — Generally low GI, low-GL, high in antioxidants, carb content: low to moderate. Acai berries are celebrated for their profound antioxidant levels and fiber, which aid in heart health and digestion.
- **Acerola (all fresh, frozen, dried fruits or 100% fruit juices)** — Low GI, very high in vitamin C, carb content: low.

Acerola cherries are an exceptional source of vitamin C, enhancing immune function and skin health.

- **Apricots (all fresh, frozen, dried fruits or 100% fruit juices)** — Low GI, especially when fresh. High in vitamins A and C, and a good source of fiber, carb content: low. Apricots support vision health and immune function.
- **Asian Pears (all fresh, frozen, dried fruits or 100% fruit juices)** — Low to moderate GI, good fiber content, carb content: low. These pears offer a juicy and refreshing taste with a mild sweet flavor, beneficial for hydration and satiety.
- **Avocados (all fresh, frozen, dried fruits or 100% fruit juices)** — Very low GI, high in healthy fats, carb content: very low. Avocados are also rich in fiber and vitamins C, E, K, and B-6, supporting cardiovascular health and weight management.
- **Blackberries (all fresh, frozen, dried fruits or 100% fruit juices)** — Very low GI, high in dietary fiber, vitamins C and K, and antioxidants, carb content: low. Blackberries contribute to heart health and cancer prevention.
- **Blueberries (all fresh, frozen, dried fruits or 100% fruit juices)** — Low to moderate GI, rich in antioxidants and fiber, carb content: low. Blueberries are known for enhancing brain health and reducing the risk of diabetes.
- **Boysenberry (all fresh, frozen, dried fruits or 100% fruit juices)** — Low GI, high in fiber and vitamins, carb content: moderate. Known for their deep flavor, boysenberries aid in digestive health and sustain stable blood sugar levels.
- **Calamondin (all fresh, frozen, dried fruits or 100% fruit juices)** — Low GI, carb content: low. Rich in vitamin C, these are great for tropical flavored dishes and provide immune support.
- **Cantaloupe (all fresh, frozen, dried fruits or 100% fruit juices)** — Low to moderate GI, rich in vitamins A and C, hydrating, and has a high water content, carb content: moderate. Cantaloupe aids in skin health and hydration.

- **Cherimoya (all fresh, frozen, dried fruits or 100% fruit juices)** — Moderate GI, carb content: high. Rich in vitamin C and dietary fiber, cherimoya supports digestive health and immune function.
- **Cherries (all fresh, frozen, dried fruits or 100% fruit juices)** — Low GI, good source of fiber, vitamin C, and anthocyanins, carb content: moderate. Cherries are beneficial for joint health and sleep improvement.
- **Coconut (all fresh, frozen, dried fruits or 100% fruit juices)** — Low GI, high in medium-chain fatty acids, carb content: low. Coconut supports metabolism and provides a quick source of energy.
- **Cranberry (all fresh, frozen, dried fruits or 100% fruit juices)** — Low GI, carb content: low. Cranberries are high in vitamin C and are particularly beneficial for urinary tract health.
- **Currant (all fresh, frozen, dried fruits or 100% fruit juices)** — Low GI, carb content: moderate. Currants are rich in antioxidants and vitamin C, which support immune function and overall health.
- **Damson Plum (all fresh, frozen, dried fruits or 100% fruit juices)** — Low GI, carb content: moderate. Damson plums are a rich source of fiber and vitamins (A, C, and E), helpful for digestive health.
- **Durian (all fresh, frozen, dried fruits or 100% fruit juices)** — High GI, carb content: high. Known for its substantial fiber and vitamin content, durian should be consumed in moderation due to its higher carbohydrate content.
- **Grapefruit (all fresh, frozen, dried fruits or 100% fruit juices)** — Low GI, high in vitamin C and soluble fiber, carb content: low. Grapefruit can aid in cholesterol management and supports cardiovascular health.
- **Guava (all fresh, frozen, dried fruits or 100% fruit juices)** — Low GI, extremely rich in dietary fiber, vitamins A and C,

carb content: moderate. Guava provides more than three times the daily recommended intake of vitamin C per fruit, enhancing immune defense and skin health.

- **Honeydew Melon (all fresh, frozen, dried fruits or 100% fruit juices)** — Low GI, provides a good source of vitamin C and is hydrating with its high water content, carb content: moderate. Honeydew is ideal for hydration and providing a quick, refreshing snack.
- **Huckleberries (all fresh, frozen, dried fruits or 100% fruit juices)** — Low GI, carb content: low. Huckleberries are high in antioxidants and fiber, promoting cardiovascular health and blood sugar regulation.
- **Jujube (all fresh, frozen, dried fruits or 100% fruit juices)** — Moderate GI, carb content: high. Jujubes are known for their high vitamin C content, supporting immune health and stress reduction.
- **Kiwifruit (all fresh, frozen, dried fruits or 100% fruit juices)** — Low to moderate GI, high in vitamins C and K, and fiber, carb content: moderate. Kiwifruit aids in digestion and boosts immune system function.
- **Lemonquat (all fresh, frozen, dried fruits or 100% fruit juices)** — Low GI, carb content: low. This hybrid fruit is rich in vitamin A, B9, C and provides a tangy addition to various dishes while supporting immune health.
- **Limes (all fresh, frozen, dried fruits or 100% fruit juices)** — Low GI, carb content: low. High in vitamin B6, B9, C and antioxidants, limes are excellent for enhancing flavor in dishes without adding sugar.
- **Lychee (all fresh, frozen, dried fruits or 100% fruit juices)** — High GI, carb content: high. Rich in vitamin C, lychee should be consumed in the recommended serving size due to its high sugar content.
- **Mangoes (all fresh, frozen, dried fruits or 100% fruit juices)** — Low GI (54), high in carbohydrates. Mangoes are

abundant in vitamins A, B6, C, and fiber, which help supporting immune function and digestive health.

- **Mulberries (all fresh, frozen, dried fruits or 100% fruit juices)** — Low GI, moderate carbohydrate content. They are rich in vitamins C, B6, K, manganese and iron, beneficial for maintaining healthy blood and antioxidant levels.
- **Nectarines (all fresh, frozen, dried fruits or 100% fruit juices)** — Low GI, moderate carbohydrate content. Nectarines are a good source of vitamins A, C, E and K similar to peaches, and are great for skin health and immune support.
- **Olives (all fresh, frozen, dried fruits or 100% fruit juices)** — Low GI, low in carbohydrates but high in healthy fats, particularly oleic acid, which is good for heart health.
- **Oranges (all fresh, frozen, dried fruits or 100% fruit juices)** — Moderate GI, rich in vitamin C, potassium, and fiber, with a moderate carbohydrate content. Oranges support immune health and aid in digestive wellness.
- **Papaya (all fresh, frozen, dried fruits or 100% fruit juices)** — Moderate GI, rich in vitamins A, C, and E. High in fiber and water content, making it excellent for hydration and digestive health, with moderate carbohydrate content.
- **Peaches (all fresh, frozen, dried fruits or 100% fruit juices)** — Low GI when fresh, containing vitamins A and C along with fiber. The carbohydrate content ranges from low to moderate, supporting overall health without spiking blood sugar levels.
- **Pears (all fresh, frozen, dried fruits or 100% fruit juices)** — Low GI, high in fiber which assists in gradual sugar absorption, with moderate carbohydrate content. Pears help maintain steady blood sugar levels.
- **Persimmon (all fresh, frozen, dried fruits or 100% fruit juices)** — Moderate to high GI, high in carbohydrates. They are rich in fiber and vitamins, promoting digestive health and providing nutritional benefits.
- **Pineapple (all fresh, frozen, dried fruits or 100% fruit

juices) — Medium GI, but rich in vitamins C and manganese, with high carbohydrate content. Pineapple is great for immune support and antioxidant protection.

- **Plums (all fresh, frozen, dried fruits or 100% fruit juices)** — Low GI, moderate carbohydrate content. When dried (prunes), they retain their fiber and nutrients, aiding in blood sugar control and digestive health.
- **Pomegranate (all fresh, frozen, dried fruits or 100% fruit juices)** — Moderate GI, high in antioxidants and vitamins, with moderate carbohydrate content. Pomegranate helps improve heart health and reduces inflammation.
- **Raspberries (all fresh, frozen, dried fruits or 100% fruit juices)** — Very low GI, low in carbohydrates, high in dietary fiber, vitamins C, and manganese. Raspberries are excellent for maintaining stable blood sugar and providing antioxidant protection.
- **Rhubarb (all fresh, frozen, dried fruits or 100% fruit juices)** — Low GI, low carbohydrate content. Known for its high vitamin K content, rhubarb supports bone health and blood clotting processes.
- **Sapote (all fresh, frozen, dried fruits or 100% fruit juices)** — Moderate GI, moderate carbohydrate content. High in vitamin B6, C, and E.
- **Soursop (all fresh, frozen, dried fruits or 100% fruit juices)** — Moderate GI, moderate carbohydrate content. Known for its unique flavor and high vitamins and minerals content, soursop is good for immune support and cellular health.
- **Strawberries (all fresh, frozen, dried fruits or 100% fruit juices)** — Low GI, high in fiber, vitamins C, and manganese, with low carbohydrate content. Strawberries support heart health and blood sugar control.
- **Tangerines (Mandarins) (all fresh, frozen, dried fruits or 100% fruit juices)** — Low to moderate GI, low-GL. Thangerines are good source of vitamins (A, C, B6, thiamin,

folate) and fiber, with moderate carbohydrate content. Tangerines contribute to immune defense and digestive health.

- **Watermelon (all fresh, frozen, dried fruits or 100% fruit juices)** — Despite its high GI, watermelon has a low glycemic load due to its high water content, rich in vitamins (A, B6, C, folate) with moderate carbohydrate content. Watermelon is excellent for hydration and providing essential nutrients.

21

THE GRAINS DIABETES-FRIENDLY FOOD LISTS

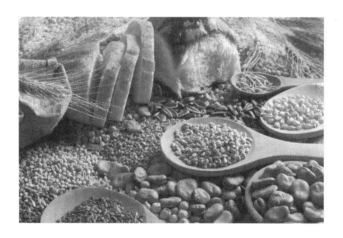

Grains in the Low glycemic Load (GL) Diabetes Diet

Aligned with MyPlate.gov's classification, the grains group includes all types of grains, such as whole grains (e.g., whole wheat, brown rice, quinoa) and refined grains (e.g., white rice, white flour). For those following a low-GL diabetes diet, the focus is primarily on whole grains, which generally have lower GL values and provide a richer nutrient profile, making them preferable for daily consumption.

Nutrient Density and Benefits of Whole Grains:

Whole grains are densely packed with nutrients, providing abundant vital nutrients while maintaining a low-calorie content. They are excellent sources of:

- **Complex Carbohydrates and Dietary Fibers:** Slowly digested, these help sustain stable blood sugar levels and enhance satiety.
- **B Vitamins:** These nutrients are crucial for a range of metabolic functions, such as generating energy and forming red blood cells.
- **Minerals:** Including iron for blood health, magnesium for muscle and nerve function, and selenium for immune support.

Experts recommend incorporating at least three servings of whole grains daily, equating to about 15-20 grams of total carbohydrates or 15 grams of net carbohydrates, consistent with low-GL diabetes diet recommendations.

CALCULATED PORTION SIZES FOR VARIOUS WHOLE GRAINS

To meet these dietary guidelines, the following portion sizes are recommended:

- **Porridge Oats**: 23 to 30 grams
- **Muesli**: 25 to 30 grams
- **Toasted Whole Grain Oat Cereal**: 20 to 27 grams
- **Multi-grain Bread**: 1 slice (31 to 42 grams per slice)
- **Brown Rice**: 65 to 87 grams (cooked)
- **Wholewheat Pasta**: 60 to 80 grams (cooked)
- **Wholewheat Bread**: 1 slice (33 to 44 grams per slice)
- **Rye Bread**: 1 slice (31 to 42 grams per slice)

- **Barley Bread**: 1 slice (33 to 44 grams per slice, similar to wholewheat bread)
- **Bran Cereal**: 23 to 31 grams
- **Cooked Cereal (e.g., wheat, oats)**: 75 to 100 grams (cooked)
- **Barley**: 54 to 71 grams (cooked)
- **Buckwheat**: 75 to 100 grams (cooked)
- **Quinoa**: 71 to 95 grams (cooked)
- **Amaranth**: 65 to 87 grams (cooked)
- **Teff**: 75 to 100 grams (cooked)
- **Bulgur**: 83 to 111 grams (cooked)
- **Sorghum**: 60 to 80 grams (cooked)
- **Millet**: 65 to 87 grams (cooked)
- **Wild Rice**: 71 to 95 grams (cooked)
- **Triticale**: 75 to 100 grams (cooked)

Whole Grains and Diabetes Management:

Evidence strongly supports the inclusion of whole grains in the low-GL Diabetes Diet as an effective strategy for diabetes management. Regular consumption of whole grains, especially types like oats known for their positive effects on glycemic markers, is crucial for controlling diabetes and enhancing overall health.

Studies show that whole grains can improve insulin sensitivity and reduce blood sugar levels post-meals. Diets rich in whole grains significantly improve markers such as fasting blood glucose, fasting insulin, glycated hemoglobin (HbA1c), and insulin resistance, especially when compared to diets high in refined grains or low in whole grains.

Research Highlights on Whole Grains:

Whole Grains and Diabetes Prevention: Higher intake of whole grains is linked to improved sensitivity and enhanced postprandial blood glucose levels.

Specific Whole Grains: Different whole grains, like oats, brown rice, and whole wheat, have specific impacts on glycemic control. Oats, in particular, are noted for their significantly beneficial effects on glycemic markers.

Mechanisms: The benefits of whole grains are thought to stem from their high fiber content, which slows glucose absorption and lowers post-meal blood glucose and insulin levels. Additionally, whole grains contain bioactive compounds that may improve insulin sensitivity.

Quantity and Frequency: The positive effects of whole grains on glycemic control are dose-dependent; greater intakes are linked with more significant improvements. Regular consumption is recommended for sustained benefits.

CRITIQUES OF THE "FREE GRAIN DIET" FOR DIABETES:

Nutritional Deficiencies: Whole grains are a significant source of nutrients like dietary fiber, B vitamins, and minerals. Eliminating them might lead to deficiencies, requiring careful planning or supplementation.

Fiber Intake: A diet without whole grains may result in insufficient fiber intake, which is crucial for digestive health and blood sugar regulation.

Impact on Gut Health: Grain fibers act as prebiotics, supporting gut bacteria health. Reducing these can negatively affect gut microbiome diversity and overall health.

Unsustainability and Restrictiveness: Completely avoiding grains can be unsustainable and may foster an unhealthy relationship with food.

Overemphasis on Elimination: Focusing solely on grain elimination overlooks the importance of a balanced diet, which should include a variety of foods for effective diabetes management.

Lack of Long-term Evidence: There is limited research on the long-term impacts of completely grain-free diets on diabetes management.

Individual Variability: Responses to grain consumption can vary significantly among individuals with diabetes.

THE LOW-GL DIABETES DIET LIST

Here is a detailed list of whole grains and pseudo-grains with an emphasis on ensuring each recommended serving size contains about 15 grams of carbohydrates, typically aligning with a low-GL:

Whole Grains

- **Barley** — Low-GL for the recommended serving size, which provides substantial fiber aiding in slow-GLucose absorption.
- **Brown Rice** — Low to moderate GL, when portioned correctly, supports steady energy with its complex carbohydrates.
- **Bulgur** — Low-GL at proper serving sizes, known for quick preparation and maintaining blood sugar levels.
- **Millet** — Naturally gluten-free with a low-GL, offers versatile uses in a diabetic diet.
- **Oats (Avena sativa L.)** — Low-GL, especially when consumed as steel-cut or old-fashioned oats, beneficial for heart and glycemic health.
- **Dark Rye** — Low-GL when eaten in appropriate portions, denser and more filling which helps in managing hunger and blood sugar.
- **Whole Wheat Bread** — Moderate GL, selecting high-fiber varieties ensures better glycemic control.
- **Whole Wheat Chapati** — Moderate GL, provides sustained energy release when eaten in controlled amounts.

- **Whole Grain Cereals** — The GL varies; choosing less processed options with no added sugars keeps the GL low.
- **Wild Rice** — Low-GL, offers a nutritious alternative to traditional white rice with more protein and fiber.
- **Sorghum** — Low-GL, this versatile, gluten-free grain can be popped like popcorn or used as a rice substitute.
- **Triticale** — Low to moderate GL, combines the qualities of wheat and rye for a nutrient-rich grain choice.
- **Pseudo-grains**
- **Buckwheat** — Low-GL, provides a hearty, nutritious option for breakfast porridge or as a rice substitute.
- **Quinoa** — Low-GL for the recommended serving, complete protein that's ideal for vegetarian diets.
- **Amaranth** — Low-GL, this protein-rich pseudo-grain is excellent for porridge or added to soups and stews.
- **Spelt** — Moderate GL, spelt offers a nutty flavor and can replace wheat in most recipes.
- **Kamut** — Low-GL, known for its rich, buttery flavor and higher protein content compared to regular wheat.
- **Teff** — Low-GL, highly nutritious, ideal for making porridge or gluten-free baked goods.

These grains and pseudo-grains should be incorporated into meals in measured amounts to maintain a low-GL, supporting effective diabetes management through controlled blood sugar levels. Each grain can contribute to a balanced diet, enhancing overall health while providing essential nutrients and energy.

22

THE DAIRY AND PLANT-BASED ALTERNATIVES DIABETES-FRIENDLY FOOD LISTS

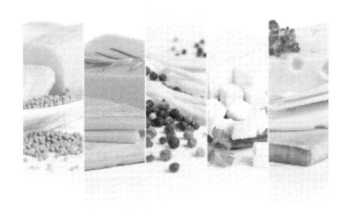

The Dairy and Plant-Based Alternatives Group in the Low-GL Diabetes Diet

Aligned with MyPlate.gov's classification, the dairy group includes all forms of dairy products such as milk, cheese, yogurt, and butter, as well as plant-based alternatives like almond milk, soy milk, and coconut yogurt. For those on the low-GL diabetes diet, the focus is on selecting options that are low in added sugars and high in calcium and other essential nutrients.

NUTRIENT DENSITY AND BENEFITS OF DAIRY AND PLANT-BASED ALTERNATIVES

Dairy products and their plant-based alternatives can be nutrient-rich, providing essential nutrients with varying calorie contents. They serve as excellent sources of calcium, vitamin D, and protein, providing added health advantages.

- **Calcium and Vitamin D**: Crucial for bone health, these nutrients help prevent osteoporosis and support muscle function.
- **Protein**: Essential for adequate muscle repair and growth, protein also helps regulate blood sugar by slowing the digestion of carbohydrates.
- **Probiotics**: Present in fermented dairy products such as yogurt and kefir, probiotics support digestive health and can enhance immune function.

Choices in the Dairy and Plant-Based Alternatives Group:

Milk and Milk Alternatives: Choose unsweetened versions of soy, almond, and oat milk, which are low-GL and rich in vitamins and minerals.

Cheese: Opt for natural cheeses which are low in carbohydrates but should be consumed in moderation due to their high saturated fat content.

Yogurt: Unsweetened, plain yogurt, particularly Greek yogurt, is recommended for its low carbohydrate content and high protein level.

Butter and Cream: These contain minimal carbohydrates but are high in saturated fats and should be used sparingly.

Dairy and Smoothies: Incorporating dairy or plant-based milk and yogurt into smoothies can enhance nutritional intake and help achieve a balanced macronutrient profile, which is beneficial for stabilizing blood glucose levels. Adding healthy fats, such as avocado or nuts, can further enrich the nutritional value of these smoothies.

PORTION SIZES AND INTAKE RECOMMENDATIONS:

For those with diabetes, it is crucial to manage the intake of dairy and dairy alternatives effectively, as even small amounts of added sugars can influence blood sugar levels. Portion control is key to minimizing impact on glucose levels:

- **Carbohydrate Management:** Aim for each serving to contain less than 12 grams of carbohydrates, especially important for milk and yogurt.
- **Daily Recommendations:** It is generally advised for adults to incorporate 3 servings of dairy or plant-based alternatives daily as part of a balanced diet. This helps ensure an adequate intake of essential nutrients while maintaining blood sugar control.

Here's a table summarizing the serving sizes for dairy and plant-based alternatives, each designed to align with low-GL recommendations and diabetes management goals:

Product Type	Recommended Serving Size	Carbohydrate Content
Unsweetened Soy Milk	1 cup	3-4 grams
Unsweetened Almond Milk	1 cup	1-2 grams
Unsweetened Oat Milk	1 cup	15-19 grams
Plain Greek Yogurt	1/2 cup	5-7 grams
Natural Cheese	1 ounce	0-1 grams
Tofu	1/2 cup (cubed)	1-2 grams
Soy Yogurt (unsweetened)	1/2 cup	4-6 grams
Cottage Cheese	1/2 cup	4-5 grams

Recommendations for Dairy and Plant-Based Alternatives in Diabetes Management

To effectively incorporate dairy and plant-based alternatives into a low-GL diabetes diet, consider the following strategies:

- **Select Minimally Processed Options:** Choose unsweetened and additive-free dairy and plant-based alternatives to minimize carbohydrate content, which is essential for maintaining a low-GL diet.
- **Diversify Your Choices:** Use a variety of non-dairy milks such as unsweetened soy, almond, and oat milk, each offering unique nutritional benefits. For instance, soy milk is high in protein, aiding in blood sugar control.
- **Focus on Probiotic-Rich Foods:** Opt for plain, unsweetened yogurts that contain probiotics, such as yogurt and soy yogurt. Probiotics are beneficial for digestive health and can

positively influence the balance of gut flora, aiding diabetes management.

- **Adhere to Recommended Portions:** Carefully measure servings, particularly for products like oat milk which may have higher carbohydrate contents, to ensure control over carbohydrate intake and stable blood glucose levels.
- **Incorporate Healthy Proteins:** Include low-carbohydrate, protein-rich foods like tofu and cottage cheese in your diet. These can be versatile in various dishes, contributing to satiety and muscle maintenance without causing blood sugar spikes.
- **Use in Balanced Meals:** Integrate dairy and plant-based alternatives thoughtfully into meals. For example, blend soy milk into smoothies, add tofu to stir-fries, or enjoy Greek yogurt with nuts and seeds for a balanced snack.

Implementing these recommendations helps ensure that each dietary choice not only supports blood sugar control but also contributes to overall health.

THE LOW-GL DIABETES DIET FOOD LIST

Here's a detailed breakdown of dairy and plant-based alternatives suitable for the low-GL diabetes diet:

Dairy and Plant-Based Milk Alternatives

- **Cow's Milk** — Available in fluid, evaporated, or dry forms, including lactose-free and reduced options. Cow's milk provides significant amounts of calcium, vitamin D, and protein but can vary in carbohydrate content depending on the type (whole, skim, etc.).

- **Goat's Milk** — Similar to cow's milk in nutrient profile, goat's milk provides a good alternative for those looking for different flavor profiles or digestibility. It is also available in lactose-free forms.
- **Buttermilk**—Traditionally left over after churning butter, it is now commercially produced as cultured buttermilk. It is lower in fat and calories but high in potassium and calcium and available in lactose-reduced forms.
- **Soy Milk** — A plant-based milk alternative without added sugars or additives, rich in protein and fortified with calcium and vitamins typically found in cow's milk. It has a low GI and is a good option for those avoiding dairy.
- **Almond Milk**—Made from ground almonds and water, this milk alternative is low in calories and carbohydrates, making it suitable for a low-GL diet when unsweetened.
- **Coconut Milk**—Extracted from the flesh of coconuts, this milk is rich in medium-chain triglycerides (MCTs) and usually low in carbohydrates, making it suitable for a low-GL diet when unsweetened.
- **Oat Milk** — Derived from whole oat grains, it's higher in carbohydrates than some other plant-based milk but offers a good amount of fiber and is often enriched with vitamins and minerals.
- **Cashew Milk** — Similar to almond milk, cashew milk is low in carbohydrates and calories, provided it's unsweetened, making it a viable option for those monitoring their blood sugar levels.
- **Rice Milk** — Generally the highest in carbohydrates among plant milks, unsweetened rice milk can still be part of a diabetes diet if portion sizes are controlled.

Dairy and Fermented Products

- **Yogurt** — Including Greek, Bulgarian, and plain varieties, without added sugars. Rich in protein and probiotics, these yogurts support digestive health and can aid manage blood sugar levels.

- **Kefir**—A fermented milk drink similar to thin yogurt, kefir is high in probiotics and low in lactose. It is excellent for gut health and potentially beneficial for blood sugar control.
- **Frozen Yogurt** — Often enjoyed as a dessert, choose versions without added sugars and watch portions to ensure they fit within the low-GL eating pattern (15 grams of carbs at most).

Cheese Varieties

- **Cheeses**—Including natural, low-fat, and non-dairy options such as soy cheese, cheeses are generally low in carbohydrates, making them a good choice for a low-GL diet.
- **Cottage Cheese** — Low-fat versions are high in protein and low in fat, making them suitable for those managing diabetes.
- **Cream Cheese** — Low-fat and lactose-reduced varieties offer a way to enjoy this spread without significantly impacting blood sugar levels.
- **Ricotta Cheese** — Typically used in sweet and savory dishes, ricotta can be part of a diabetes-friendly diet when choosing low-fat and lactose-reduced options.

Plant-Based Proteins

- **Soy Cheese** — A non-dairy alternative low in carbohydrates and can be used similarly to dairy cheese.
- **Tempeh** — Made from fermented soybeans, tempeh is high in protein and fiber, which are beneficial for blood sugar management.
- **Tofu**—Also derived from soy, tofu is characterized by its low carbs content and high protein content, making it a favorable option for individuals following a low glycemic load diet.

This detailed list offers a variety of dairy—and plant-based alternatives, providing options to enjoy while ensuring they maintain balanced blood sugar levels.

23

PROTEIN DIABETESDIABETES-FRIENDLY FOOD LISTS

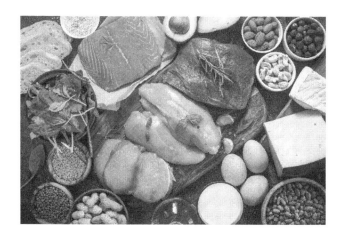

The Protein Foods Group in the Low-GL Diabetes Diet

Aligned with MyPlate.gov's classification, the protein foods group includes a diverse array of both animal and plant-based sources such as meats, poultry, fish, eggs, nuts, seeds, and legumes. For those following a low glycemic Load (GL) diabetes diet, selecting lean, minimally processed protein sources is crucial. These options should provide essential nutrients without unnecessary additives or high levels of saturated fats.

Incorporating Protein Foods into Meals: Protein enhances flavor and satiety and helps maintain stable blood glucose levels. When combined with carbohydrates, protein can delay the absorption of sugar into the bloodstream, preventing spikes.

NUTRIENT DENSITY AND BENEFITS OF PROTEIN FOODS

Protein foods are crucial for a balanced diet, offering more than just protein but also a variety of vital vitamins, minerals, and other beneficial compounds:

- **High-Quality Protein**: Essential for muscle repair, growth, and overall health. Protein also helps regulate blood sugar levels by promoting satiety and slowing the digestion of carbohydrates.
- **Omega-3** : Present in fatty fish such as salmon, mackerel, and sardines, omega-3s help reduce inflammation and are linked to heart health.
- **Iron and Zinc**: Meat, especially red meat, is a significant source of iron and zinc, which are vital for immune function and energy metabolism.
- **Fiber and Phytonutrients**: Plant-based proteins such as beans, lentils, and chickpeas offer fiber, which helps manage blood sugar levels, and phytonutrients that play a role in reducing chronic disease risk.

Choices in the Protein Foods Group:

Lean Meats: Choose options like chicken, turkey, and lean cuts of beef and pork. Prefer cooking methods like grilling, baking, or steaming without added fats or sugars.

Fish and Seafood: Focus on fatty fish for added omega-3 fatty acids. Opt for fresh or frozen varieties prepared with minimal added fats.

Eggs: A versatile source, eggs can be incorporated into a range of dishes from omelets to salads.

Legumes: Beans, chickpeas, and lentils are excellent for fiber-rich protein options that are especially beneficial in a diabetes diet.

Nuts and Seeds: Include a variety such as cashews, walnuts, almonds, flaxseeds, and chia seeds for their protein, healthy fats, and fiber.

Plant-Based Proteins: Foods like tofu, tempeh, and edamame provide high-quality protein and other nutrients beneficial for diabetes management.

PORTION SIZES AND INTAKE RECOMMENDATIONS:

Managing protein intake is essential for individuals with diabetes, particularly to avoid excessive saturated fat intake. Optimal serving sizes ensure a balanced nutrient intake without overloading on calories:

Protein Management: Aim for approximately 15-25 grams of protein per meal, tailored to individual dietary needs and total daily calorie intake.

Daily Recommendations: Adults should generally include 2-3 servings of lean protein sources each day as part of a balanced diet, ensuring they meet their target dietary protein intake as detailed in the chapter "Protein — The Building Blocks of Life."

By focusing on high-quality, minimally processed protein sources and balancing intake, individuals following a low-GL diet can effectively manage diabetes and support overall health.

Here's a table summarizing the serving sizes for protein foods with nutritional informations:

Protein Source	Serving Size	Key Nutrients	Specific Notes
Poultry (Chicken, Turkey)	3-4 ounces	Protein, B vitamins	Ideal for general health and muscle maintenance
Fish (Salmon, Tuna, Mackerel)	3-4 ounces	Protein, omega-3 fatty acids	Supports heart health and reduces inflammation
Seafood (Shrimp, Crabs)	3-4 ounces	Protein, essential minerals	Low in fat and calories
Lean Beef	3-4 ounces	Protein, iron, zinc	Choose lean cuts to reduce intake of saturated fats
Legumes (Beans, Lentils)	1/2 cup cooked	Protein, fiber, iron	Great plant-based protein source, helps in blood sugar control
Nuts and Seeds (Almonds, Walnuts, Flaxseeds)	1/4 cup	Protein, healthy fats, fiber	Enhances satiety, good for heart health
Tofu	1/2 cup	Protein, calcium	Plant-based, suitable for those managing CKD
Eggs	1-2 eggs	Protein, vitamins D and B12	Versatile and nutrient-dense
Dairy (Cheese, Yogurt)	1 ounce (cheese), 1/2 cup (yogurt)	Protein, calcium, probiotics	Choose low-fat and unsweetened varieties for diabetes management
Plant-Based Alternatives (Tempeh, Seitan)	3-4 ounces	Protein	Suitable for vegans and those with dietary restrictions

THE LOW-GL DIABETES DIET FOOD LIST

Meats, Poultry, Eggs, and Seafood Group: This group is an essential part of the diet, offering high-quality protein and vital nutrients that are crucial for health. Here's how each type can be integrated into a low glycemic Load (GL) diabetes diet:

- **Beef, Lamb, Pork, Goat**: Choose lean cuts (e.g., sirloin, tenderloin) and prefer grass-fed options when possible. These meats should be consumed in moderation and cooked adequately to preserve nutrients and ensure safety. Ground versions should be at least 90% lean.

- **Game Meat (Bison, Venison, Elk, Moose)**: Naturally leaner, these meats are abundant sources of protein and iron. They should be cooked thoroughly to optimize digestibility and safety.

- **Chicken and Turkey**: Skinless options are preferred to minimize fat intake. Both can be enjoyed cooked adequately in various forms, such as roasted, grilled, or boiled. Ground chicken or turkey should be considered if it's at least 93% lean.
- **Duck and Goose**: Higher in fat, these should be consumed less frequently and with the skin removed to reduce fat content.
- **Game Birds (Ostrich, Pheasant, Quail)**: These are excellent sources of lean protein and should be cooked thoroughly to ensure safety.

- **Chicken, Duck, Turkey, and Other Birds' Eggs**: Eggs are versatile and can be consumed cooked in styles such as boiled, scrambled, or poached. They provide high-quality protein, important vitamins and minerals.

Seafood

- **Fatty Fish (Salmon, Mackerel, Sardines, Herring, Trout)**: Rich in omega-3 fatty acids, these should be included regularly in the diet. They can be consumed cooked adequately through methods like grilling or baking.
- **White Fish (Cod, Tilapia, Flounder, Sole, Pollock)**: Low in fat and high in protein, ideal for frequent consumption cooked adequately to maintain nutrient integrity.
- **Shellfish (Shrimp, Lobster, Crab, Clams, Oysters, Scallops)**: High in protein and minerals but should be consumed in

moderation due to cholesterol content. Ensure they are cooked thoroughly to avoid foodborne illnesses.

- **Other Seafood (Squid, Octopus)**: These can be included and should be cooked adequately to ensure they are tender and safe to eat.

Nuts, Seeds, and Soy Products in the Low-GL Diabetes Diet

This group is essential for providing healthy fats, proteins, fiber, and various micronutrients that can enhance overall health and help manage diabetes more effectively.

Nuts and Nut Butter

Nuts are a heart-healthy food group rich in unsaturated fats, proteins, vitamins, and minerals. They can be incorporated into the low-GL diabetes diet in moderation due to their high caloric content:

- **Almonds**: High in vitamin E and magnesium, helpful for blood sugar control.
- **Pecans**: Rich in antioxidants and beneficial fats.
- **Brazil Nuts**: Best known for their selenium content, which supports thyroid function.
- **Pistachios**: Good for heart health, with a balance of protein and fiber.
- **Hazelnuts**: High in vitamin E and healthy fats.
- **Macadamias**: High in monounsaturated fats.
- **Pine Nuts**: Good source of iron and magnesium.
- **Walnuts**: Rich in alpha-linolenic acid, an omega-3 fatty acid.
- **Cashew Nuts**: Lower fat content than other nuts, rich in copper and magnesium.

Nut butter should be chosen carefully, ensuring it is natural and without added sugars or excessive salts.

Seeds and Seed Butter

Seeds offer similar nutritional benefits as nuts but are generally higher in fiber and contain unique beneficial compounds:

- **Pumpkin Seeds**: A good magnesium, zinc, and fatty acids source.
- **Psyllium Seeds**: These are mainly used for their fiber content, which can help digestion and aid stabilize blood sugar levels.
- **Chia Seeds**: Exceptionally high in omega-3 and fiber.
- **Flax Seeds**: High in omega-3 and lignans, which have antioxidant properties.
- **Sunflower Seeds**: Rich in vitamin B6, E, thiamine and selenium.
- **Sesame Seeds**: Good source of calcium and magnesium.
- **Poppy Seeds**: Contain calcium, iron, and zinc.

Like nut butter, seed butter (e.g., sunflower butter or tahini, made from sesame seeds) should be chosen without added sugars or salts and can be used in various culinary applications, from dressings to spreads.

Soy Products

Soy products are excellent plant-based protein sources that can be beneficial in a diabetes diet:

- **Tofu**: Versatile and can be used in savory and sweet dishes; high in protein and calcium when fortified.
- **Tempeh**: Fermented, making it richer in protein and nutrients than tofu and easier to digest.
- **Edamame**: Young soybeans are often eaten as a snack; high in protein and fiber.
- **Soy Milk**: An alternative option to dairy milk; choose unsweetened varieties to keep sugar intake low.

Integration into the Diet

Nuts, seeds, and soy products can be incorporated into the diet in various ways:

- **As a Snack**: Raw or roasted nuts and seeds are great for snacking.
- **In Meals**: Add nuts or seeds to salads, yogurt, or oatmeal for extra texture and nutrients.
- **Soy Products**: Use tofu in stir-fries, soups, and stews, or blend silken tofu into smoothies for added protein.

THE GI, GL & NET CARB COUNTER

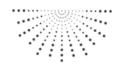

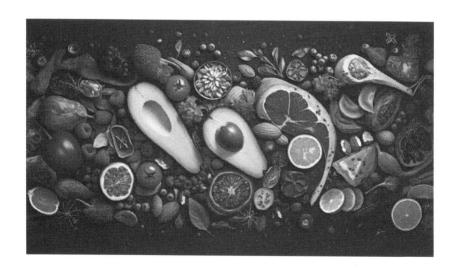

INTRODUCTION TO THE GLYCEMIC INDEX AND GLYCEMIC LOAD COUNTER

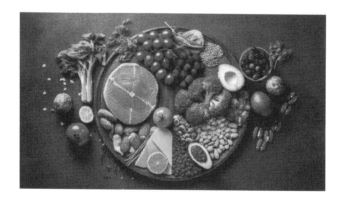

INTRODUCTION TO THE GI, GL & NET CARB COUNTER FOR THE LOW-GL DIABETES DIET

The GI, GL, and Net Carb counter is a critical tool for implementing fully the Low-GL Diabetes Diet in your daily meal planning. This counter differs from others by focusing exclusively on foods that are appropriate for diabetes management, avoiding highly processed foods, those high in advanced glycation end-products (AGEs), sodium, or cholesterol.

Selection and Evaluation Process: We started with an initial list of over 4,000 foods, applying stringent criteria based on the principles of a Low glycemic Load (GL) Diabetes Diet. Our selection process involved excluding foods that were inherently unsuitable for a diabetes-friendly diet—particularly those high in processed content, added sugars, sodium, and unhealthy fats, or prepared through non-compliant methods such as frying and breading. This meticulous vetting reduced the list to 1,100 items, removing over 2,900 choices that were either irrelevant or potentially harmful for diabetes management.

Understanding Food Suitability: The suitability of foods in this counter depends on their Glycemic Load (GL). We aim to provide detailed information about each "potentially diabetes-friendly" food, including its Glycemic Index (GI), Glycemic Load (GL), net carbohydrate content, and recommended serving sizes. The term "potentially" is crucial here, indicating that our evaluations provide nuanced insights beyond simple classifications like "whole food" or "minimally processed food."

Counter Structure: The counter is organized into 12 primary food categories to simplify navigation and selection:

- Breads and Baked Products
- Beans & Lentils
- Beverages
- Dairy Products
- Dairy Alternatives — Plant-based Options
- Dressings & Oils
- Fruits
- Fruit Products
- Grains, Cereals, Pasta & Rice
- Herbs and Spices
- Nuts & Seeds
- Vegetables & Vegetable Products

This structure allows users to quickly locate and choose healthy options within each essential food group.

Using the Counter:

- **Select From Food Groups:** Start with any MyPlate.gov food groups such as fruits, vegetables, grains, proteins, and dairy. Items within the 12 categories are listed alphabetically for easy reference.
- **Prioritize Glycemic Load (GL):** Focus on foods classified as having a low glycemic Load (GL) for your daily diet. Foods with a medium GL, ranging between 10 and 19, can occasionally be included to diversify your dietary choices without significantly impacting your blood sugar levels.
- **Adapt the Serving Sizes:** It's crucial to adjust the counter's specified serving sizes to maintain net carbohydrates under 15 grams per serving, essential for managing carbohydrate intake effectively.
- **Choose Low-GL Options:** When selecting within a food subcategory, opt for the item with the lowest GL. Understanding the direct physiological impact of GL values is vital: 1 GL unit is equivalent to the effect of consuming 1 gram of pure glucose.
- **Balance Your Diet:** In addition to focusing on GL and net carbs, it's important to maintain a balanced diet. Incorporate a variety of foods from all categories to fulfill overall nutritional requirements, reinforcing the dietary guidelines and meal planning principles introduced earlier.

By presenting a streamlined selection, this counter aims to simplify dietary decision-making and support efficient and confident diabetes management.

2

BREADS AND BAKED PRODUCTS

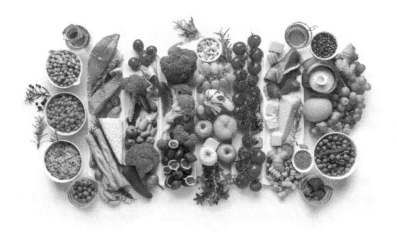

BAKED FOODS & BREADS	SERVING SIZE	NET CARB (g)	GI VALUE	GI LEVEL	GL VALUE	GL LEVEL
Almond Flour Bread	1 slice, 25g	3	35	Low	1.1	Low
Apple Pie	1 slice, 125g	32	70	High	22.4	High
Apple Turnover	1 med., 100g	33	45	Low	14.9	Med.
Bacon Cheddar Biscuits	1 biscuit, 64g	25	70	High	17.5	Med.
Baguette	1 serv., 50g	25	95	High	23.8	High
Bakewell Tart	1 slice, 80g	35	76	High	26.6	High
Baklava	1 piece, 33g	29	85	High	24.7	High
Bannock	1 piece, 60g	24	77	High	18.5	Med.
Barley Bread	1 slice, 25g	12	34	Low	4.1	Med.
Beignets	1 med., 60g	34	81	High	27.5	High
Biscotti	1 biscotti, 20g	12	70	High	8.4	Low
Biscuit Sandwiches	1 sandwich, 130g	28	70	High	19.6	High
Black Forest Cake	1 slice, 100g	34	74	High	25.2	High
Black Forest Tart	1 slice, 100g	25	76	High	19	Med.

BAKED FOODS & BREADS	SERVING SIZE	NET CARB (g)	GI VALUE	GI LEVEL	GL VALUE	GL LEVEL
Blackberry Pie	1 slice, 125g	29	70	High	20.3	High
Blueberry Custard Tart	1 slice, 100g	21	76	High	16	Med.
Blueberry pie	1 slice, 125g	30	70	High	21	High
Boston Cream Pie	1 slice, 100g	34	70	High	23.8	High
Brioche	1 slice, 30g	15	82	High	12.3	Med.
Buckwheat Bread	1 slice, 25g	15	47	Low	7.1	Low
Butter Cookies	1 cookie, 30g	11	73	High	8	Low
Buttermilk Biscuits	1 biscuit, 64g	24	70	High	16.8	Med.
Buttermilk Pie	1 slice, 125g	38	70	High	26.6	High
Cannoli	1 med., 85g	32	75	High	24	High
Carrot Cake	1 slice, 100g	40	74	High	29.6	High
Challah	1 slice, 40g	20	78	High	15.6	Med.
Cheese and Herb Biscuits	1 biscuit, 35g	13	70	High	9.1	Low
CheeseCake	1 slice, 100g	28	74	High	20.7	High
Cherry Pie	1 slice, 125g	31	70	High	21.7	High

BAKED FOODS & BREADS	SERVING SIZE	NET CARB (g)	GI VALUE	GI LEVEL	GL VALUE	GL LEVEL
Chocolate Cake	1 slice, 100g	35	74	High	25.9	High
Chocolate Chip Biscuits	1 biscuit, 57g	33	70	High	23.1	High
Chocolate Chip Cookies	1 cookie, 30g	19	73	High	13.9	Med.
Chocolate Pecan Pie	1 slice, 125g	42	70	High	29.4	High
Chocolate Silk Pie	1 slice, 100g	26	70	High	18.2	Med.
Chocolate Tart	1 slice, 100g	23	76	High	17.5	Med.
Churros	1 med., 30g	24	82	High	19.7	High
Ciabatta	1 serv., 50g	20	78	High	15.6	Med.
Cinnamon Roll	1 small, 60g	31	82	High	25.4	High
Cinnamon Roll Biscuits	1 biscuit, 28g	20	70	High	14	Med.
Coconut Cake	1 slice, 80g	31	74	High	22.9	High
Coconut Cream Pie	1 slice, 100g	26	70	High	18.2	Med.
Coconut Flour Bread	1 slice, 25g	2	45	Low	0.9	Low
Coconut Macaroons	1 macaroon, 20g	10	75	High	7.5	Low

BAKED FOODS & BREADS	SERVING SIZE	NET CARB (g)	GI VALUE	GI LEVEL	GL VALUE	GL LEVEL
Coffee Cake	1 slice, 100g	38	74	High	28.1	High
Corn Tortilla	1 med., 55g	13	70	High	9.1	Low
Cornbread	1 piece, 60g	28	65	Med.	18.2	Med.
Cornish Pasty	1 small, 150g	40	83	High	33.2	High
Croissant	1 med.,57g	23	81	High	18.6	Med.
Custard Tart	1 slice, 100g	20	76	High	15.2	Med.
Danish Pastry	1 med., 84g	37	85	High	31.5	High
Dobos Torte	1 slice, 100g	31	81	High	25.1	High
Double Chocolate Cookies	1 cookie, 30g	19	73	High	13.9	Med.
Drop Biscuits	1 biscuit, 30g	11	70	High	7.7	Low
Eccles Cake	1 Cake, 60g	27	74	High	20	High
Éclair	1 med., 85g	26	88	High	22.9	High
Empanada	1 small, 100g	35	75	High	26.3	High
Ezekiel Bread	1 slice, 25g	12	36	Low	4.3	Low
Flaxseed Bread	1 slice, 25g	10	45	Low	4.5	Low

BAKED FOODS & BREADS	SERVING SIZE	NET CARB (g)	GI VALUE	GI LEVEL	GL VALUE	GL LEVEL
Focaccia	1 slice, 50g	20	72	High	14.4	Med.
Fougasse	1 serv., 50g	20	71	High	14.2	Med.
French Bread	1 slice, 30g	15	95	High	14.3	Med.
Garlic Butter Biscuits	1 biscuit, 25g	10	70	High	7	Low
German Chocolate Cake	1 slice, 100g	38	74	High	28.1	High
Gingerbread Cookies	1 cookie, 30g	16	73	High	11.7	Med.
Gluten-Free Multiseed Bread	1 slice, 25g	11	55	Low	6.1	Low
Green Onion Biscuits	1 biscuit, 28g	14	70	High	9.8	Low
Ham and Cheese Biscuits	1 biscuit, 60g	20	70	High	14	Med.
Hummingbird Cake	1 slice, 80g	37	74	High	27.4	High
Irish Soda Bread	1 slice, 45g	20	65	Med.	13	Med.
Italian Bread	1 slice, 30g	14	70	High	9.8	Low
Keto Bread	2 slice, 50g	4	10	Low	0.4	Low
Lemon Cake	1 slice, 100g	31	74	High	22.9	High
Lemon Cookies	1 cookie, 30g	14	73	High	10.2	Med.
Lemon Meringue Pie	1 slice, 125g	31	70	High	21.7	High

BAKED FOODS & BREADS	SERVING SIZE	NET CARB (g)	GI VALUE	GI LEVEL	GL VALUE	GL LEVEL
Lemon Mousse Tart	1 slice, 100g	22	76	High	16.7	Med.
Linzer Cookies	1 cookie, 30g	16	73	High	11.7	Med.
Low-Carb Tortilla	1 med., 55g	6	30	Low	1.8	Low
Marble Cake	1 slice, 100g	36	74	High	26.6	High
Mille Crepe Cake	1 slice, 100g	33	74	High	24.4	High
Mississippi Mud Pie	1 slice, 100g	30	70	High	21	High
Mixed Berry Pie	1 slice, 100g	18	70	High	12.6	Med.
Molasses Cookies	1 cookie, 30g	17	73	High	12.4	Med.
Naan	1 piece, 60g	26	81	High	21.1	High
Oat Bread	1 slice, 25g	15	66	Med.	9.9	Low
Oatmeal Raisin Cookies	1 cookie, 30g	16	69	Med.	11	Med.
Orange Cake	1 slice, 80g	31	74	High	22.9	High
Panettone	1 slice, 50g	23	72	High	16.6	Med.
Pão de Queijo	1 piece, 30g	15	75	High	11.3	Med.
Peach Pie	1 slice, 125g	27	70	High	18.9	Med.

BAKED FOODS & BREADS	SERVING SIZE	NET CARB (g)	GI VALUE	GI LEVEL	GL VALUE	GL LEVEL
Peanut Butter Blossoms	1 cookie, 30g	13	76	High	9.9	Low
Peanut Butter Cookies	1 cookie, 30g	13	73	High	9.5	Low
Pecan Pie	1 slice, 125g	41	70	High	28.7	High
Pesto Biscuits	1 biscuit, 28g	15	70	High	10.5	Med.
Pita Bread	1 small pita, 35g	18	81	High	14.6	Med.
Pithivier	1 small, 90g	36	88	High	31.7	High
Pound Cake	1 slice, 100g	37	74	High	27.4	High
Pretzel	1 med., 60g	22	75	High	16.5	Med.
Puff Pastry	1 sheet, 79g	36	84	High	30.2	High
Pumpernickel Bread	1 slice, 25g	13	53	Low	6.9	Low
Pumpkin Biscuits	1 biscuit, 28g	15	70	High	10.5	Med.
Pumpkin Pie	1 slice, 125g	30	70	High	21	High
Quiche	1 slice, 100g	10	75	High	7.5	Low
Quinoa Bread	1 slice, 25g	13	30	Low	3.9	Low

BAKED FOODS & BREADS	SERVING SIZE	NET CARB (g)	GI VALUE	GI LEVEL	GL VALUE	GL LEVEL
Raspberry Tart	1 slice, 100g	15	76	High	11.4	Med.
Rhubarb Pie	1 slice, 125g	26	70	High	18.2	Med.
Rosemary Biscuits	1 biscuit, 38g	15	70	High	10.5	Med.
Rye Bread	1 slice, 25g	14	62	Med.	8.7	Low
Shortbread Cookies	1 cookie, 30g	11	73	High	8	Low
Simit	1 piece, 60g	22	78	High	17.2	Med.
Snickerdoodle Cookies	1 cookie , 30g	14	73	High	10.2	Med.
Sourdough Bread	1 slice, 25g	15	65	Med.	9.8	Low
Soy and Linseed Bread	1 slice, 25g	10	55	Low	5.5	Low
Spelt Bread	1 slice, 25g	16	53	Low	8.5	Low
Sponge Cake	1 slice, 100g	33	74	High	24.4	High
Strawberry ShortCake	1 slice, 100g	32	74	High	23.7	High
Strawberry Tart	1 biscuit, 50g	22	76	High	16.7	Med.
Strudel	1 slice, 100g	41	81	High	33.2	High
Sweet Potato Biscuits	1 cookie, 30g	16	70	High	11.2	Med.

BAKED FOODS & BREADS	SERVING SIZE	NET CARB (g)	GI VALUE	GI LEVEL	GL VALUE	GL LEVEL
Tiramisu	1 small, 60g	28	88	High	24.6	High
Tomato Tart	1 slice, 100g	30	76	High	22.8	High
Tres Leches Cake	1 slice, 100g	10	74	High	7.4	Low
Vanilla Cake	1 slice, 100g	42	74	High	31.1	High
Vol-au-vent	1 slice, 100g	34	82	High	27.9	High
Wheat Tortilla	1 med., 55g	18	70	High	12.6	Med.
Whole Grain Bread	1 slice, 25g	12	68	Med.	8.2	Low
Whole Grain Ciabatta	1 small, 25g	15	68	Med.	10.2	Med.
Whole Wheat Bread	1 slice, 30g	14	71	High	9.9	Low

3

BEANS & LENTILS

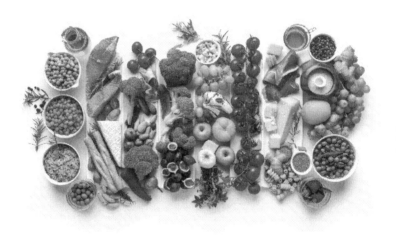

FOOD	SERVING SIZE	NET CARB (g)	GI VALUE	GI LEVEL	GL VALUE	GL LEVEL
Adzuki Bean Flour	¼ cup, 30g	18	32	Low	5.8	Low
Adzuki Bean Sprout Powder	¼ cup, 30g	14	15	Low	2.1	Low
Alfalfa Sprout Powder	¼ cup, 30g	5	15	Low	0.8	Low
Amaranth Sprout Powder	¼ cup, 30g	20	35	Low	7	Low
Azuki Bean Flour	¼ cup, 30g	18.9	33	Low	6.2	Low
Baby lima beans	½ cup, 100g	13	32	Low	6	Low
Barley Sprout Powder	¼ cup, 30g	18	25	Low	4.5	Low
Beans, fava, in pod, raw	1 cup, 130g	7.8	30	Low	2	Low
Beans, kidney, mature seeds, soaked and cooked	1 cup, 104g	3.7	40	Low	3	Low
Beans, navy, mature seeds, soaked and cooked	1 cup, 104g	2.8	30	Low	1	Low
Beans, pinto, mature seeds, soaked and cooked	1 cup, 104g	5.5	40	Low	2	Low
Beans, snap, green, soaked and cooked	1 cup, 100g	3.9	30	Low	1	Low
Beans, snap, yellow, , soaked and cooked	1 cup, 100g	3.2	30	Low	1	Low

FOOD	SERVING SIZE	NET CARB (g)	GI VALUE	GI LEVEL	GL VALUE	GL LEVEL
Black Bean Flour	¼ cup, 30g	10.5	30	Low	3.2	Low
Black beans	½ cup, 100g	13	30	Low	5	Low
Black Beans	1 cup, 172g	24	30	Low	8	Low
Black Eyed Pea Flour	¼ cup, 30g	18.9	42	Low	7.9	Low
Black turtle beans	½ cup, 100g	13	30	Low	5	Low
Black-eyed peas	½ cup, 100g	19	41	Low	8	Low
Broad Bean Flour (Fava Bean Flour)	¼ cup, 30g	17.4	79	High	13.7	Medium
Broccoli Sprout Powder	¼ cup, 30g	8	15	Low	1.2	Low
Buckwheat Sprout Powder	¼ cup, 30g	20	45	Low	9	Low
Butter Bean Flour (Lima Bean Flour)	¼ cup, 30g	18	31	Low	5.6	Low
Cabbage Sprout Powder	¼ cup, 30g	8	15	Low	1.2	Low
Cannellini Bean Flour	¼ cup, 30g	18	31	Low	5.6	Low
Cannellini beans	½ cup, 100g	13	31	Low	4	Low
Chia Sprout Powder	¼ cup, 30g	4	15	Low	0.6	Low

FOOD	SERVING SIZE	NET CARB (g)	GI VALUE	GI LEVEL	GL VALUE	GL LEVEL
Chickpea Flour (Besan)	¼ cup, 30g	13.2	44	Low	5.8	Low
Chickpeas	½ cup, 82g	13.5	28	Low	4	Low
Chickpeas, garbanzo beans	½ cup, 100g	16	28	Low	6	Low
Clover Sprout Powder	¼ cup, 30g	5	15	Low	0.8	Low
Cowpeas	½ cup, 100g	18	29	Low	7	Low
Cowpeas, leafy tips, raw	1 cup, 36g	1	20	Low	1	Low
Cowpeas, young pods with seeds, raw	1 cup, 100g	8	40	Low	4	Low
Cranberry Bean Flour	¼ cup, 30g	18	29	Low	5.2	Low
Dragon's tongue beans	½ cup, 100g	5	31	Low	2	Low
Fava Bean Flour	¼ cup, 30g	17.4	79	High	13.7	Medium
Fava beans	½ cup, 100g	13	32	Low	7	Low
Flageolet beans	½ cup, 100g	14	31	Low	4	Low
French Green Lentil Flour	¼ cup, 30g	18	28	Low	5	Low
Garbanzo Bean Flour (Gram Flour)	¼ cup, 30g	17.4	28	Low	4.9	Low

FOOD	SERVING SIZE	NET CARB (g)	GI VALUE	GI LEVEL	GL VALUE	GL LEVEL
Garlic Sprout Powder	¼ cup, 30g	14	15	Low	2.1	Low
Great Northern Bean Flour	¼ cup, 30g	18	36	Low	6.5	Low
Great Northern Beans	½ cup, 100g	15	31	Low	5	Low
Green Pea Flour	¼ cup, 30g	18	48	Low	8.6	Low
Green peas	½ cup, 100g	9	42	Low	4	Low
Kale Sprout Powder	¼ cup, 30g	8	15	Low	1.2	Low
Kidney Bean Flour	¼ cup, 30g	18	24	Low	4.3	Low
Kidney beans	½ cup, 100g	16	29	Low	7	Low
Lentil Flour	¼ cup, 30g	15	29	Low	4.4	Low
Lentil Sprout Powder	¼ cup, 30g	15	25	Low	3.8	Low
Lentils	½ cup, 100g	12	29	Low	5	Low
Lima bean flour	½ cup, 100g	19	32	Low	4	Low
Lima Bean Flour	¼ cup, 30g	18	32	Low	5.8	Low
Lima beans	½ cup, 100g	20	32	Low	8	Low

FOOD	SERVING SIZE	NET CARB (g)	GI VALUE	GI LEVEL	GL VALUE	GL LEVEL
Moth Bean Flour	¼ cup, 30g	18.9	29	Low	5.5	Low
Mung Bean Flour	¼ cup, 30g	18.9	25	Low	4.7	Low
Mung Bean Sprout Powder	¼ cup, 30g	12	15	Low	1.8	Low
Mung beans	½ cup, 100g	12	32	Low	4	Low
Navy Bean Flour	¼ cup, 30g	18	38	Low	6.8	Low
Navy beans	½ cup, 100g	11	31	Low	3.5	Low
Pea Sprout Powder	¼ cup, 30g	14	15	Low	2.1	Low
Peanuts	1 oz, 28g	3	33	Low	1	Low
Pinto Bean Flour	¼ cup, 30g	18	39	Low	7	Low
Quinoa Sprout Powder	¼ cup, 30g	20	35	Low	7	Low
Radish Sprout Powder	¼ cup, 30g	5	15	Low	0.8	Low
Red beans	½ cup, 100g	15	35	Low	5.3	Low
Red kidney beans	½ cup, 100g	13	40	Low	7	Low
Red Lentil Flour	¼ cup, 30g	18	26	Low	4.7	Low

FOOD	SERVING SIZE	NET CARB (g)	GI VALUE	GI LEVEL	GL VALUE	GL LEVEL
Red lentils	½ cup, 100g	13	44	Low	8	Low
Soy Flour	¼ cup, 30g	6	15	Low	0.9	Low
Soybean Sprout Powder	¼ cup, 30g	8	15	Low	1.2	Low
Soybeans	½ cup, 100g	10	33	Low	6	Low
Split peas	½ cup, 100g	12	32	Low	5	Low
Sunflower Sprout Powder	¼ cup, 30g	8	15	Low	1.2	Low
Wheatgrass Sprout Powder	¼ cup, 30g	15	15	Low	2.3	Low
White Bean Flour	¼ cup, 30g	18	31	Low	5.6	Low
White beans	½ cup, 100g	12	45	Low	7	Low
Yellow Split Pea Flour	¼ cup, 30g	18	35	Low	6.3	Low

4

BEVERAGES

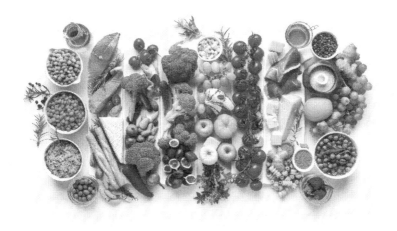

BEVERAGES & DRINKS	SERVING SIZE	NET CARB (g)	GI VALUE	GI LEVEL	GL VALUE	GL LEVEL
Apple Cider Vinegar - diluted as beverage-	1 cup, 240ml	0	0	Low	0	Low
Beer	1 cup, 240ml	8	50	Low	4	Low
Beer Birch	1 cup, 240ml	34	68	Med.	23.1	High
Beer light	1 cup, 240ml	4	50	Low	2	Low
Beer Root	1 cup, 240ml	30	63	Med.	18.9	Med.
Beet Kvass	1 cup, 240ml	10	60	Med.	6	Low
Café au lait	1 cup, 240ml	4	30	Low	1.2	Low
Caffè Breve	1 cup, 240ml	4	50	Low	2	Low
Caffè Corretto	1 cup, 240ml	0	0	Low	0	Low
Caffè Mocha	1 cup, 240ml	32	50	Low	16	Med.
Cappuccino	1 cup, 240ml	8	50	Low	4	Low
Caramel Latte	1 cup, 240ml	25	50	Low	12.5	Med.
Caramel Macchiato	1 cup, 240ml	25	50	Low	12.5	Med.

BEVERAGES & DRINKS	SERVING SIZE	NET CARB (g)	GI VALUE	GI LEVEL	GL VALUE	GL LEVEL
Carbonated Lemonade	1 cup, 240ml	30	72	High	21.6	High
Carbonated Water with Natural Flavors	1 cup, 240ml	0	0	Low	0	Low
Coconut Water	1 cup, 240ml	9	35	Low	3.2	Low
Coffee Espresso	¼ cup, 60ml	0	0	Low	0	Low
Coffee Iced/Hot	1 cup, 240ml	0	0	Low	0	Low
Cola Soda regular	1 cup, 240ml	26	63	Med.	16.4	Med.
Cortado	4 fl oz, 120g	0	0	Low	0	Low
Cream Soda	1 cup, 240ml	30	71	High	21.3	High
Diet Cola	1 cup, 240ml	0	0	Low	0	Low
Diet Lemon-Lime Soda	1 cup, 240ml	0	0	Low	0	Low
Electrolyte Water	1 cup, 240ml	0	0	Low	0	Low
Energy Drink regular	1 cup, 240ml	28	72	High	20.2	High
Energy Drink sugar-free	1 cup, 240ml	0	0	Low	0	Low
Energy Shot	1 cup, 240ml	30	70	High	21	High

BEVERAGES & DRINKS	SERVING SIZE	NET CARB (g)	GI VALUE	GI LEVEL	GL VALUE	GL LEVEL
Frappuccino	1 cup, 240ml	50	50	Low	25	High
Fruit Punch	1 cup, 240ml	28	67	Med.	18.8	Med.
Ginger Ale	1 cup, 240ml	26	63	Med.	16.4	Med.
Grape Soda	1 cup, 240ml	40	63	Med.	25.2	High
Horchata	1 cup, 240ml	43	70	High	30.1	High
Hot Apple Toddy	1 cup, 240ml	10	0	Low	0	Low
Hot Chocolate	1 cup, 240ml	30	60	Med.	18	Med.
Hot Chocolate with Whipped Cream	1 cup, 240ml	35	63	Med.	22.1	High
Iced Chai Tea Latte	1 cup, 240ml	25	50	Low	12.5	Med.
Isotonic Beverage	1 cup, 240ml	10	50	Low	5	Low
Kombucha	1 cup, 240ml	2	10	Low	0.2	Low
Kvass	1 cup, 240ml	7	40	Low	2.8	Low
Lactose-Free Protein Drink	1 cup, 240ml	3	30	Low	0.9	Low
Lassi Low-carb Drink	1 cup, 240ml	10	30	Low	3	Low

BEVERAGES & DRINKS	SERVING SIZE	NET CARB (g)	GI VALUE	GI LEVEL	GL VALUE	GL LEVEL
Latte Macchiato	1 cup, 240ml	10	40	Low	4	Low
Lemon-Lime Soda	1 cup, 240ml	26	63	Med.	16.4	Med.
Macchiato	1 cup, 240ml	10	40	Low	4	Low
Malt Drink	1 cup, 240ml	35	50	Low	17.5	Med.
Malted Milk	1 cup, 240ml	45	50	Low	22.5	High
Matcha Green Tea Iced/Hot	1 cup, 240ml	0	0	Low	0	Low
Milk Chocolate	1 cup, 240ml	23	60	Med.	13.8	Med.
Orange Soda Regular	1 cup, 240ml	28	72	High	20.2	High
Post-workout Recovery Drink	1 cup, 240ml	25	50	Low	12.5	Med.
Protein Shake	1 cup, 240ml	5	25	Low	1.3	Low
Protein Shake Whey Based	1 cup, 240ml	7	30	Low	2.1	Low
Pumpkin Spice Latte	1 cup, 240ml	52	70	High	36.4	High
Red Soda regular	1 cup, 240ml	31	63	Med.	19.5	High
Rice Wine	5 fl oz, 100g	3	10	Low	0.3	Low

BEVERAGES & DRINKS	SERVING SIZE	NET CARB (g)	GI VALUE	GI LEVEL	GL VALUE	GL LEVEL
Rum	1 fl oz, 30g	0	0	Low	0	Low
Sake	5 fl oz, 100g	1	20	Low	0.2	Low
Sarsaparilla	1 cup, 240ml	25	50	Low	12.5	Med.
Smoothie Chocolate Banana	1 cup, 240ml	68	45	Low	30.6	High
Sparkling Water	1 cup, 240ml	0	0	Low	0	Low
Stevia-Sweetened Soda	1 cup, 240ml	0	0	Low	0	Low
Tea Black/Green	1 cup, 240ml	0	0	Low	0	Low
Tea Bubble	1 cup, 240ml	60	70	High	42	High
Tea Chai /Chamomile /Ginger /Mint	1 cup, 240ml	0	0	Low	0	Low
Tea Herbal	1 cup, 240ml	0	0	Low	0	Low
Tea Thai Iced	1 cup, 240ml	25	50	Low	12.5	Med.
Tepache	1 cup, 240ml	25	55	Low	13.8	Med.
Tequila	1 fl oz, 30g	0	0	Low	0	Low
Tonic Water	1 cup, 240ml	25	50	Low	12.5	Med.

BEVERAGES & DRINKS	SERVING SIZE	NET CARB (g)	GI VALUE	GI LEVEL	GL VALUE	GL LEVEL
Turmeric Latte	1 cup, 240ml	14	40	Low	5.6	Low
Vinegar -diluted as a beverage-	1 cup, 240ml	0	0	Low	0	Low
Vodka	1 fl oz, 30g	0	0	Low	0	Low
Whiskey	1 fl oz, 30g	0	0	Low	0	Low
Wine Mulled	5 fl oz, 148g	15	50	Low	7.5	Low
Wine red	5 fl oz, 148g	2.7	0	Low	0	Low
Wine white	5 fl oz, 148g	2.8	0	Low	0	Low

5

DAIRY PRODUCTS

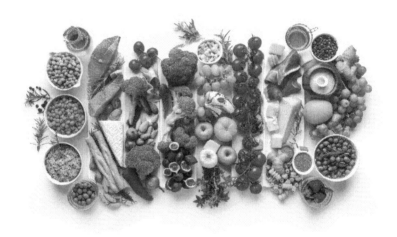

FOOD	SERVING SIZE	NET CARB (g)	GI VALUE	GI LEVEL	GL VALUE	GL LEVEL
American Cheese	1 oz, 28g	2	0	Low	0	Low
Appenzeller	1 oz, 28g	0.1	1-10	Low	0	Low
Asiago	1 oz, 28g	0.9	1-10	Low	0	Low
Blue cheese	1 oz, 28g	0.7	1-10	Low	0	Low
Brie Cheese	1 oz, 28g	1	0	Low	0	Low
Burrata	1 oz, 28g	1	1-10	Low	0.1	Low
Butter	1 tbsp, 14g	0	0	Low	0	Low
Buttermilk	1 cup, 245g	12	46	Low	5.5	Low
Camembert	1 oz, 28g	0.1	1-10	Low	0	Low
Cheddar	1 oz, 28g	0.4	1-10	Low	0.1	Low
Chèvre	1 oz, 28g	0.2	1-10	Low	0.1	Low
Colby Cheese	1 oz, 28g	0	0	Low	0	Low
Colby Jack Cheese	1 oz, 28g	1	0	Low	0	Low
Comté	1 oz, 28g	0.4	1-10	Low	0.1	Low
Cottage Cheese	1 cup, 226g	6	10	Low	0.6	Low
Cottage Cheese Flavored	1 cup, 226g	15	10	Low	1.5	Low
Cottage Cheese Large Curd	1 cup, 240g	10	10	Low	1	Low

FOOD	SERVING SIZE	NET CARB (g)	GI VALUE	GI LEVEL	GL VALUE	GL LEVEL
Cottage Cheese Low-fat	1 cup, 226g	6	10	Low	0.6	Low
Cottage Cheese Non-fat	1 cup, 226g	10	10	Low	1	Low
Cottage Cheese Small Curd	1 cup, 240g	10	10	Low	1	Low
Cream Cheese	1 oz, 28g	1	0	Low	0	Low
Cream Cheese Flavored	1 oz, 28g	2	0	Low	0	Low
Cream Cheese Low-fat	1 oz, 28g	1	0	Low	0	Low
Cream Cheese Non-fat	1 oz, 28g	2	0	Low	0	Low
Cream Cheese Spread	1 tbsp, 14g	1	0	Low	0	Low
Creamer Dairy-based	1 tbsp, 15ml	5	47	Low	2.4	Low
Edam Cheese	1 oz, 28g	1	0	Low	0	Low
Emmental	1 oz, 28g	0.4	1-10	Low	0.1	Low
Farmer Cheese	1 cup, 226g	10	10	Low	1	Low
Feta	1 oz, 28g	1.2	1-10	Low	0.1	Low
Fontina	1 oz, 28g	0.4	1-10	Low	0.1	Low
Ghee (Clarified Butter)	1 tbsp, 14g	0	0	Low	0	Low
Goat Cheese	1 oz, 28g	1	0	Low	0	Low
Gorgonzola	1 oz, 28g	0.3	1-10	Low	0.1	Low

FOOD	SERVING SIZE	NET CARB (g)	GI VALUE	GI LEVEL	GL VALUE	GL LEVEL
Gouda Cheese	1 oz, 28g	1	0	Low	0	Low
Gruyere Cheese	1 oz, 28g	0	0	Low	0	Low
Half and Half	1 tbsp, 15ml	0	0	Low	0	Low
Halloumi	1 oz, 28g	1	1-10	Low	0.1	Low
Havarti Cheese	1 oz, 28g	1	0	Low	0	Low
Heavy Cream	1 tbsp, 15ml	0	0	Low	0	Low
Hot Mocha	1 cup, 240ml	30	50	Low	15	Med.
Hot Peppermint Mocha	1 cup, 240ml	30	50	Low	15	Med.
Iced Chai Tea Latte	1 cup, 240ml	25	50	Low	12.5	Med.
Kefir	1 cup, 240g	12	20	Low	2.4	Low
Labneh	1 oz, 28g	2	0	Low	0	Low
Limburger Cheese	1 oz, 28g	0	0	Low	0	Low
Manchego	1 oz, 28g	0	1-10	Low	0	Low
Mascarpone	1 oz, 28g	1	0	Low	0	Low
Milk Chocolate	1 cup, 240ml	23	60	Med.	13.8	Med.
Milk Lactose-free	1 cup, 244g	12	27-45	Low	5.4	Low

FOOD	SERVING SIZE	NET CARB (g)	GI VALUE	GI LEVEL	GL VALUE	GL LEVEL
Milk Organic	1 cup, 244g	12	27-45	Low	5.4	Low
Milk Skim	1 cup, 244g	12	27-45	Low	5.4	Low
Milk Whole	1 cup, 244g	12	27-45	Low	5.4	Low
Monterey Jack	1 oz, 28g	0.5	1-10	Low	0.1	Low
Monterey Jack Cheese	1 oz, 28g	1	0	Low	0	Low
Monterey Jack with Jalapeño	1 oz, 28g	0.4	1-10	Low	0.1	Low
Mozzarella	1 oz, 28g	0.6	1-10	Low	0.1	Low
Mozzarella Cheese	1 oz, 28g	1	0	Low	0	Low
Muenster	1 oz, 28g	0.3	1-10	Low	0.1	Low
Neufchâtel Cheese	1 oz, 28g	1	0	Low	0	Low
Panela Cheese	1 oz, 28g	0	0	Low	0	Low
Parmesan	1 oz, 28g	0.9	1-10	Low	0.1	Low
Pecorino Romano	1 oz, 28g	0.5	1-10	Low	0.1	Low
Pepper Jack	1 oz, 28g	0.5	1-10	Low	0.1	Low
Provolone Cheese	1 oz, 28g	1	0	Low	0	Low
Provolone piccante	1 oz, 28g	0.6	1-10	Low	0.1	Low
Quark	1 cup, 225g	9	0	Low	0	Low
Queso Blanco	1 oz, 28g	0	0	Low	0	Low

FOOD	SERVING SIZE	NET CARB (g)	GI VALUE	GI LEVEL	GL VALUE	GL LEVEL
Queso de Bola -Edam Cheese-	1 oz, 28g	0	0	Low	0	Low
Queso Fresco	1 oz, 28g	0	0	Low	0	Low
Ricotta Cheese	1 cup, 246g	11	10	Low	1.1	Low
Ricotta Salata	1/4 cup, 62g	3	1-10	Low	0.3	Low
Romano Cheese	1 oz, 28g	0	0	Low	0	Low
Sarsaparilla	1 cup, 240ml	25	50	Low	12.5	Med.
Sour Cream	1 cup, 230g	15	14	Low	2.1	Low
Sour Cream, Low-fat	Low-fat	10	14	Low	1.4	Low
Stilton Cheese	1 oz, 28g	0.4	1-10	Low	0.1	Low
Swiss Cheese	1 oz, 28g	2	1-10	Low	0.2	Low
Taleggio	1 oz, 28g	0.1	1-10	Low	0.1	Low
Whipped Butter	1 tbsp, 14g	0	0	Low	0	Low
Whipped Cream	1 cup, 240g	10	0	Low	0	Low
Whipped Topping	1 cup, 120g	10	0	Low	0	Low
Yogurt Greek Full-fat	1 cup, 227g	10	11	Low	1.1	Low
Yogurt Greek Low-fat	1 cup, 227g	10	11	Low	1.1	Low

FOOD	SERVING SIZE	NET CARB (g)	GI VALUE	GI LEVEL	GL VALUE	GL LEVEL
Yogurt Greek Low-fat	1 cup, 245g	10	11	Low	1.1	Low
Yogurt Greek Non-fat	1 cup, 227g	10	11	Low	1.1	Low
Yogurt Greek Non-fat	1 cup, 245g	10	11	Low	1.1	Low
Yogurt Greek Non-fat Greek	1 cup, 227g	10	11	Low	1.1	Low
Yogurt Greek Plain	1 cup, 227g	10	11	Low	1.1	Low
Yogurt Greek Plain	1 cup, 245g	10	11	Low	1.1	Low
Yogurt Greek Whole Milk	1 cup, 227g	10	11	Low	1.1	Low
Yogurt Smoothie	1 cup, 240ml	30	50	Low	15	Med.

6

DAIRY ALTERNATIVES — PLANT-BASED OPTIONS

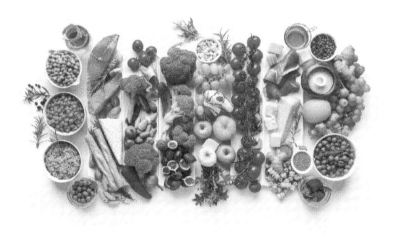

FOOD	SERVING SIZE	NET CARB (g)	GI VALUE	GI LEVEL	GL VALUE	GL LEVEL
Almond milk yogurt	1 cont., 150g	4	10	Low	0.4	Low
Almond milk	1 cup, 240 ml	2	30	Low	0.6	Low
Cashew milk yogurt	1 cont., 150g	7	10	Low	0.7	Low
Cashew milk	1 cup, 240 ml	4	30	Low	1.2	Low
Coconut milk yogurt	1 cont., 150g	15	50	Low	7.5	Low
Coconut Milk	1 cup, 240ml	21	50	Low	10.5	High
Creamer Non-dairy	1 tbsp, 15ml	4	34	Low	1.4	Low
Extra Firm Tofu	½ cup, 126g	2	15	Low	0.3	Low
Firm Tofu	½ cup, 126g	2	15	Low	0.3	Low
Flax milk	1 cup, 240 ml	1	10	Low	0.1	Low
Hazelnut milk	1 cup, 240 ml	19.9	50	Low	0.2	Low
Hemp milk	1 cup, 240 ml	2	20	Low	0.4	Low
Macadamia Milk	1 cup, 240ml	3	35	Low	1.1	Low

FOOD	SERVING SIZE	NET CARB (g)	GI VALUE	GI LEVEL	GL VALUE	GL LEVEL
Oat Milk	1 cup, 240ml	21	69	Med.	14.6	Med.
Pea milk	1 cup, 240 ml	2	34	Low	0.7	Low
Pistachio Milk	1 cup, 240ml	5	35	Low	1.8	Low
Post-workout Recovery Drink	1 cup, 240ml	25	50	Low	12.5	Med.
Pre-workout Energy Drink	1 cup, 240ml	30	65	Med.	19.5	Med.
Rice Milk	1 cup, 250ml	26	86	High	22.4	High
Quinoa Milk	1 cup, 240ml	8	54	Low	1.8	Low
Silken Tofu	½ cup, 126g	1	15	Low	0.2	Low
Soy Butter	1 tbsp, 14g	0	0	Low	0	Low
Soy Cheese	1 oz, 28g	0	14	Low	0	Low
Soy Cottage Cheese	1 cup, 240g	5	15	Low	0.8	Low
Soy Cream Cheese	1 oz, 28g	0	14	Low	0	Low
Soy Creamer	1 tbsp, 15ml	2	34	Low	0.7	Low
Soy Milk, Plain	Plain	4	34	Low	1.4	Low
Soy Milk	1 cup, 240ml	10	34	Low	3.4	Low

FOOD	SERVING SIZE	NET CARB (g)	GI VALUE	GI LEVEL	GL VALUE	GL LEVEL
Soy Protein Powder	1 scoop, 30g	2	25	Low	0.5	Low
Soy Ricotta Cheese	1 cup, 246g	4	15	Low	0.6	Low
Soy Sour Cream	1 tbsp, 14g	2	18	Low	0.4	Low
Soy Whipped Topping	1 tbsp, 5g	0	0	Low	0	Low
Soy Yogurt, Plain	1 cont., 150g	15	32	Low	4.8	Low
Soy-based Coffee Creamer	1 tbsp, 15ml	6	34	Low	0.7	Low
Soy-based Creamer	1 tbsp, 15ml	2	34	Low	0.7	Low
Soy-based Desserts	1 serv., 100g	2	34	Low	5.1	Low
Soy-based Milkshake	1 cup, 240ml	15	34	Low	5.1	Low
Soy-based Whipped Cream	1 tbsp, 5g	15	0	Low	0	Low
Sports Drinks	1 cup, 240ml	0	60	Med.	18	Med.
Tempeh	1 cup, 166g	30	35	Low	3.5	Low
Tepache	1 cup, 240ml	10	55	Low	13.8	Med.
Tiger Nut Milk	1 cup, 240ml	25	65	Med.	15.6	Med.

FOOD	SERVING SIZE	NET CARB (g)	GI VALUE	GI LEVEL	GL VALUE	GL LEVEL
Tofu	½ cup, 126g	24	15	Low	0.2	Low
Walnut Milk	1 cup, 240ml	1	25	Low	0.3	Low

7

DRESSINGS & OILS

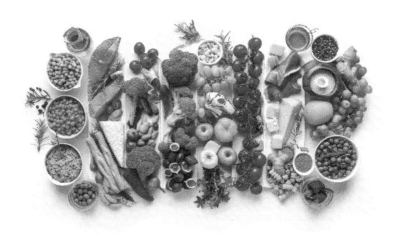

FOOD	SERVING SIZE	NET CARB (g)	GI VALUE	GI LEVEL	GL VALUE	GL LEVEL
Alfredo Sauce	¼ cup, 62 g	1.6	27	Low	0.4	Low
Beef Tallow	1 tbsp, 15 g	0	0	Low	0	Low
Clarified Butter	1 tbsp, 15 g	0	0	L	0	Low
Cocktail sauce	¼ cup, 62 g	18	38	Low	6.8	Low
Dressing, Blue or roquefort	2 tbsp, 30 g	8.1	50	Low	4.1	Low
Dressing, Blue or roquefort, low-calorie	2 tbsp, 30 g	0.9	5	Low	0	Low
Dressing, Caesar	¼ cup, 62 g	1.6	50	Low	0.8	Low
Dressing, Caesar, low-calorie	¼ cup, 62 g	0.2	5	Low	0	Low
Dressing, Coleslaw	¼ cup, 62 g	2.3	50	Low	1.2	Low
Dressing, Coleslaw, reduced calorie	¼ cup, 62 g	0	5	Low	0	Low
Dressing, Cream cheese	2 tbsp, 30 g	1	50	Low	0.5	Low
Dressing, Feta Cheese	¼ cup, 62 g	1.4	50	Low	0.7	Low
Dressing, French	2 tbsp, 30 g	9	50	Low	4.5	Low

FOOD	SERVING SIZE	NET CARB (g)	GI VALUE	GI LEVEL	GL VALUE	GL LEVEL
Dressing, French, reduced calorie	2 tbsp, 30 g	3.8	50	Low	1.9	Low
Dressing, Green Goddess	2 tbsp, 30 g	2.4	50	Low	1.2	Low
Dressing, Honey mustard	2 tbsp, 30 g	8.4	50	Low	4.2	Low
Dressing, Italian dressing	2 tbsp, 30 g	2.2	50	Low	1.1	Low
Dressing, Italian, diet or reduced calorie	2 tbsp, 30 g	0.4	5	Low	0	Low
Dressing, Italian, reduced calorie	2 tbsp, 30 g	0.4	5	Low	0	Low
Dressing, Korean	¼ cup, 62 g	3.7	50	Low	1.9	Low
Dressing, Mayonnaise-type salad	2 tbsp, 30 g	6	50	Low	3	Low
Dressing, Mayonnaise-type salad, diet	2 tbsp, 30 g	2.2	50	Low	1.1	Low
Dressing, Milk, vinegar based	2 tbsp, 30 g	1.9	50	Low	1	Low
Dressing, Peppercorn	2 tbsp, 30 g	2	50	Low	1	Low
Dressing, Poppy seed	2 tbsp, 30 g	6.2	50	Low	3.1	Low
Dressing, Russian	2 tbsp, 30 g	9.6	50	Low	4.8	Low
Dressing, Salad, common	2 tbsp, 30 g	2.8	50	Low	1.4	Low

FOOD	SERVING SIZE	NET CARB (g)	GI VALUE	GI LEVEL	GL VALUE	GL LEVEL
Dressing, Sesame	2 tbsp, 30 g	7.4	50	Low	3.7	Low
Dressing, Thousand Island Regular	2 tbsp, 30 g	2.9	50	Low	1.5	Low
Dressing, Vinegar based	2 tbsp, 30 g	1.6	50	Low	0.8	Low
Dressing, Yogurt	2 tbsp, 30 g	1.9	50	Low	1	Low
Duck Fat	2 tbsp, 30 g	0	0	Low	0	Low
Mayonnaise (mean value)	2 tbsp, 30 g	2.4	50	Low	1.2	Low
Mayonnaise, Vegan tofu	2 tbsp, 30 g	0.6	50	Low	0.3	Low
Mustard greens (mean value)	2 tbsp, 30 g	0.5	32	Low	0.2	Low
Mustard pickles	2 tbsp, 30 g	7.5	32	Low	2.4	Low
Oil, Avocado	2 tbsp, 30 g	0	0	Low	0	Low
Oil, Canola	2 tbsp, 30 g	0	0	Low	0	Low
Oil, Coconut	2 tbsp, 30 g	0	0	Low	0	Low
Oil, Corn	2 tbsp, 30 g	0	0	Low	0	Low
Oil, Extra-virgin olive	2 tbsp, 30 g	0	0	Low	0	Low

FOOD	SERVING SIZE	NET CARB (g)	GI VALUE	GI LEVEL	GL VALUE	GL LEVEL
Oil, Flaxseed	2 tbsp, 30 g	0	0	Low	0	Low
Oil, Grapeseed	2 tbsp, 30 g	0	0	Low	0	Low
Oil, Hazelnut	2 tbsp, 30 g	0	0	Low	0	Low
Oil, Hemp seed	2 tbsp, 30 g	0	0	Low	0	Low
Oil, Macadamia Nut	2 tbsp, 30 g	0	0	Low	0	Low
Oil, Olive	2 tbsp, 30 g	0	0	Low	0	Low
Oil, Palm	2 tbsp, 30 g	0	0	Low	0	Low
Oil, Peanut	2 tbsp, 30 g	0	0	Low	0	Low
Oil, Rice Bran	2 tbsp, 30 g	0	0	Low	0	Low
Oil, Sesame	2 tbsp, 30 g	0	0	Low	0	Low
Oil, Sunflower	2 tbsp, 30 g	0	0	Low	0	Low
Oil, Vegetable	2 tbsp, 30 g	0	0	Low	0	Low
Oil, Walnut	2 tbsp, 30 g	0	0	Low	0	Low
Vinegar and water dressing	2 tbsp, 30 g	0	0	Low	0	Low

8

FRUITS

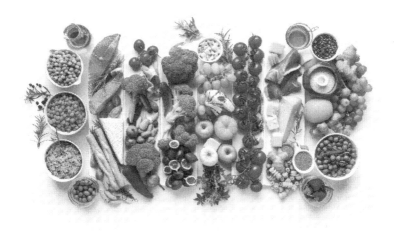

FOOD	SERVING SIZE	NET CARB (g)	GI VALUE	GI LEVEL	GL VALUE	GL LEVEL
Abiyuch	½ cup, 64g	16	45	Low	7.2	Low
Acai	½ cup, 100g	5	40	Low	2	Low
Acerola	1 cup, 98g	8	25	Low	2	Low
Ackee	½ cup, 100g	8	50	Low	4	Low
African Cherry Orange	1 fruit, 40g	4	40	Low	2	Low
African Cucumber	½ cup, 60g	4	40	Low	2	Low
Apple	1 med., 182g	21	36	Low	5	Low
Apple Kei	1 fruit, 20g	3	35	Low	1	Low
Apple Rose	1 fruit, 45g	3	30	Low	1	Low
Apple Star	1 fruit, 138g	6	35	Low	3	Low
Apple Velvet	1 fruit, 166g	9	35	Low	3	Low
Apples Golden Delicious	1 med., 174g	17	40	Low	6	Low
Apples Granny Smith	1 med., 170g	14	35	Low	5	Low
Apricot Plum	1 fruit, 50g	7	34	Low	2	Low
Asian Pears	1 med., 166g	17	35	Low	6	Low
Avocado	½ med., 100g	2	15	Low	0.3	Low

FOOD	SERVING SIZE	NET CARB (g)	GI VALUE	GI LEVEL	GL VALUE	GL LEVEL
Avocados California	½ fruit, 100g	3	20	Low	1	Low
Banana Baked	1 small, 81g	24	88	High	20.3	High
Banana extra ripe raw	1 small, 81g	22	85	High	18.7	med.
Banana ripe raw	1 small , 81g	23	75	High	16.5	med.
Banana Unripe	1 small, 81g	19	53	Low	10	Low
Barbados Cherry	½ cup, 75g	6	35	Low	2	Low
Bartlett Pears	1 med., 166g	20	35	Low	6	Low
Black Sapote	½ cup, 50g	9	35	Low	3	Low
Blackberries	1 cup, 144g	10	30	Low	3	Low
Blackberry	½ cup, 72g	7	25	Low	2	Low
Blueberries	1 cup, 148g	17	45	Low	6	Low
Blueberry	½ cup, 75g	10	40	Low	4	Low
Boysenberry	½ cup, 75g	8	30	Low	3	Low
Breadfruit	½ cup, 60g	12	60	med.	6	Low
Cantaloupe	½ cup, 89g	7	60	med.	4	Low
Cape Gooseberry	½ cup, 50g	7	40	Low	3	Low
Carissa	1 cup, 132g	18	40	Low	7	Low
Casaba Melon	1 cup, 160g	11	35	Low	4	Low

FOOD	SERVING SIZE	NET CARB (g)	GI VALUE	GI LEVEL	GL VALUE	GL LEVEL
Cempedak	½ cup, 75g	10	40	Low	4	Low
Cherimoya	½ fruit, 85g	9	35	Low	3	Low
Cherry	½ cup, 76g	10	22	Low	3	Low
Chokeberry	½ cup, 60g	6	35	Low	2	Low
Clementine	1 fruit, 74g	9	35	Low	3	Low
Cloudberry	½ cup, 60g	5	25	Low	2	Low
Coconut	½ cup, 40g	5	45	Low	2	Low
Cornelian Cherry	½ cup, 75g	6	30	Low	2	Low
Cranberry	½ cup, 50g	6	45	Low	3	Low
Currant	½ cup, 56g	8	25	Low	2	Low
Damson Plumb	½ cup, 75g	8	30	Low	3	Low
Date Plum	1 fruit, 25g	5	35	Low	2	Low
Dates	¼ cup, 40g	28	70	Low	21	High
Durian	½ cup, 100g	13	45	Low	6	Low
Elderberry	½ cup, 50g	6	25	Low	2	Low
Feijoa	1 fruit, 50g	6	35	Low	2	Low
Fig Fresh	1 med., 50g	14	60	med.	8	Low
Figs dried	¼ cup, 40g	24	61	med.	15	med.
Finger Lime	1 fruit, 10g	1	30	Low	0	Low
Gac Fruit	¼ cup, 25g	2	30	Low	1	Low

FOOD	SERVING SIZE	NET CARB (g)	GI VALUE	GI LEVEL	GL VALUE	GL LEVEL
Genip	1 fruit, 20g	3	35	Low	1	Low
Goji Berries Dried	¼ cup, 28g	17	40	Low	7.5	Low
Goldenberry	½ cup, 50g	6	35	Low	3	Low
Gooseberry	½ cup, 75g	8	25	Low	2	Low
Grape	½ cup, 75g	13	46	Low	5	Low
Grapefruit California	1 med., 154g	13	30	Low	4	Low
Graviola	½ cup, 100g	10	40	Low	4	Low
Greengage	1 fruit, 20g	3	30	Low	1	Low
Groundcherries	1 cup, 140g	20	40	Low	7	Low
Guanabana	½ cup, 100g	10	40	Low	4	Low
Guava	1 med., 55g	4	20	Low	1	Low
Hala Fruit	¼ cup, 25g	2	35	Low	1	Low
Huckleberry	½ cup, 75g	6	25	Low	2	Low
Imbe	1 fruit, 20g	2	40	Low	1	Low
Jabuticaba	½ cup, 50g	6	35	Low	3	Low
Jackfruit	½ cup, 100g	16	50	Low	8	Low
Jambul	½ cup, 75g	5	30	Low	2	Low
Jujube	1 fruit, 15g	6	50	Low	3	Low

FOOD	SERVING SIZE	NET CARB (g)	GI VALUE	GI LEVEL	GL VALUE	GL LEVEL
Kitembilla	½ cup, 50g	5	30	Low	2	Low
Kiwano	½ fruit, 100g	7	35	Low	2	Low
Kiwi	1 fruit, 69g	9	50	Low	5	Low
Kumquat	5 fruits , 50g	6	30	Low	3	Low
Langsat	½ cup, 75g	8	40	Low	3	Low
Lemon	1 fruit, 58g	3	20	Low	1	Low
Lime	1 fruit, 44g	3	20	Low	1	Low
Limequat	1 fruit, 20g	2	30	Low	1	Low
Litchis	1 cup, 190g	25	54	Low	14	med.
Loganberries	1 cup, 180g	9	30	Low	3	Low
Longan	½ cup, 50g	10	50	Low	5	Low
Loquat	½ cup, 75g	5	35	Low	2	Low
Lychee	½ cup, 75g	12	54	Low	7.1	Low
Mango	½ cup, 83g	15	54	Low	8	Low
Mango Cooked	1 cup, 165g	30	58	Low	15	med.
Mangosteen	1 fruit, 75g	6	45	Low	3	Low
Marula	1 fruit, 10g	1	30	Low	1	Low
Medlar	1 fruit, 20g	3	35	Low	1	Low
Melon	1 cup, 177g	12	65	med.	5	Low
Melon Galia	½ cup, 90g	6	65	med.	4	Low

FOOD	SERVING SIZE	NET CARB (g)	GI VALUE	GI LEVEL	GI VALUE	GL LEVEL
Melon Honeydew	½ cup, 85g	8	60	med.	4	Low
Melon Santa Claus	1 cup, 177g	13	60	med.	6	Low
Miracle Fruit	1 fruit, 5g	1	30	Low	0	Low
Mulberry	½ cup, 70g	6	25	Low	3	Low
Nance	1 cup, 120g	20	45	Low	10	Low
Nectarines	1 med., 142g	15	40	Low	6	Low
Oheloberries	1 cup, 140g	11	35	Low	5	Low
Olive	5 large, 25g	1	15	Low	0	Low
Olives Jumbo	¼ cup, 40g	1	25	Low	0	Low
Orange	1 med., 131g	12	40	Low	4	Low
Orange Mandarin	1 fruit, 88g	9	40	Low	4	Low
Orange Navel	1 med., 154g	15	40	Low	6	Low
Oranges California Valencia	1 med., 131g	14	45	Low	6	Low
Papaya	1 cup, 145g	11	60	med.	6	Low
Passion Fruit	1 fruit, 18g	2	30	Low	1	Low
Peach	1 med., 150g	10	40	Low	4	Low
Pear	1 med., 178g	21	38	Low	5	Low

FOOD	SERVING SIZE	NET CARB (g)	GI VALUE	GI LEVEL	GL VALUE	GL LEVEL
Pear Prickly	1 fruit, 103g	5	35	Low	2	Low
Persimmon	1 fruit, 25g	6	50	Low	3	Low
Pineapple	½ cup, 82g	10	59	med.	7	Low
Pitanga	1 cup, 140g	14	40	Low	7	Low
Plantain	1 cup, 148g	30	40	Low	12	Low
Plantains Cooked	½ cup, 100g	32	54	Low	17.6	med.
Plum	1 fruit, 66g	6	40	Low	2	Low
Plum Japanese	1 fruit, 40g	4	40	Low	2	Low
Pomegranate	½ cup, 87g	12	53	Low	6	Low
Pomelo	½ fruit, 154g	9	30	Low	3	Low
Prunes	¼ cup, 40g	18	29	Low	10	Low
Pummelo	1 cup, 190g	8	35	Low	4	Low
Quince	1 fruit, 92g	6	34	Low	2	Low
Raisin	¼ cup, 40g	31	66	med.	20.5	High
Raisins Golden Delicious	¼ cup, 40g	31	54	Low	17	med.
Raspberry	½ cup, 62g	3	32	Low	1	Low
Red Banana	1 med., 100g	18	45	Low	7	Low
Redcurrant	½ cup, 56g	5	25	Low	2	Low

FOOD	SERVING SIZE	NET CARB (g)	GI VALUE	GI LEVEL	GL VALUE	GL LEVEL
Rhubarb	1 cup, 122g	3	15	Low	1	Low
Sapodilla	1 fruit, 150g	14	45	Low	6	Low
Soursop	1 cup, 225g	15	45	Low	6	Low
Star Fruit	1 fruit, 91g	4	25	Low	1	Low
Strawberry	½ cup, 72g	4	32	Low	1	Low
Sweet Granadilla	1 fruit, 140g	10	40	Low	3	Low
Tahitian Pomelo	½ fruit, 154g	10	40	Low	4	Low
Tamarind	1 oz, 28g	6	40	Low	3	Low
Tangelo	1 fruit, 109g	10	42	Low	4	Low
Tangerine	1 fruit, 84g	9	40	Low	3	Low
Ugli Fruit	½ fruit, 120g	10	40	Low	4	Low
Ugni Fruit	¼ cup, 30g	4	30	Low	2	Low
Vanilla Bean	2 bean, 12g	2	50	Low	2	Low
Wampi	¼ cup, 28g	3	30	Low	1	Low
Watermelon	1 cup, 152g	11	72	High	5	Low
White Currant	½ cup, 56g	5	25	Low	2	Low
White Sapote	1 fruit, 170g	6	30	Low	2	Low

FOOD	SERVING SIZE	NET CARB (g)	GI VALUE	GI LEVEL	GL VALUE	GL LEVEL
Yellow Passion Fruit	1 fruit, 18g	2	30	Low	1	Low
Yellow Watermelon	1 cup, 152g	11	72	High	5	Low
Yuzu	1 fruit, 77g	2	30	Low	1	Low
Zante Currant	¼ cup, 40g	17	60	med.	10	Low
Ziziphus Fruit	5 fruit, 50g	15	35	Low	5.2	Low
Zombie Fruit	5 fruit, 90g	10	30	Low	5	Low

9

FRUIT PRODUCTS

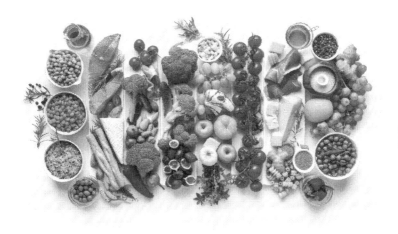

FOOD	SERVING SIZE	NET CARB (g)	GI VALUE	GI LEVEL	GL VALUE	GL LEVEL
Acerola Juice	½ cup, 120ml	6	40	Low	2.4	Low
Apple Baked Unsweetened	1 cup, 125g	23	40	Low	8	Low
Apple Butter	1 tbsp, 20g	10	45	Low	6	Low
Apple Chips	1 cup, 30g	22	50	Low	10	Low
Apple Juice	½ cup, 120ml	14	45	Low	6.3	Low
Apple Juice Concentrate	¼ cup, 60g	15	40	Low	12	med.
Apple Pickled	½ cup, 75g	12	35	Low	4	Low
Applesauce	¼ cup, 61g	12.5	40	Low	5	Low
Apricot	1 fruit, 35g	4	34	Low	2	Low
Apricot Jam Unsweetened	1 tbsp, 20g	13	54	Low	8	Low
Apricot Juice Concentrate	¼ cup, 60g	12	40	Low	6	Low
Apricots Canned Light Syrup Drained	½ cup, 122g	14	45	Low	7	Low
Beet Juice	½ cup, 120ml	11	64	med.	5	Low
Blackberries canned Light Syrup Drained	½ cup, 122g	8	25	Low	3	Low
Blackberry Jam Homemade	1 tbsp, 20g	13	54	Low	8	Low

FOOD	SERVING SIZE	NET CARB (g)	GI VALUE	GI LEVEL	GL VALUE	GL LEVEL
Blackcurrant Juice Concentrate	¼ cup, 60g	0	20	Low	0	Low
Blueberries Canned Light Syrup Drained	1 cup, 230g	23	45	Low	10	Low
Blueberries Canned Light Syrup Drained	½ cup, 122g	15	40	Low	7	Low
Blueberry Jam Homemade	1 tbsp, 20g	13	54	Low	8	Low
Blueberry Juice	½ cup, 120ml	14	40	Low	5.8	Low
Blueberry Juice Concentrate	¼ cup, 60g	12	54	Low	6.3	Low
Carrot Juice	½ cup, 120ml	9.5	43	Low	4.1	Low
Cherries Canned Light Syrup Drained	½ cup, 122g	18	60	med.	9	Low
Cherry Juice	½ cup, 120ml	14	50	Low	7	Low
Cherry Preserves	1 tbsp, 20g	13	54	Low	8	Low
Cranberry Juice	½ cup, 120ml	15	52	Low	7.5	Low
Cranberry Juice Concentrate	¼ cup, 60g	10	50	Low	5	Low
Cranberry Sauce Homemade	1 tbsp, 20g	13	54	Low	8	Low
Desert Lime	1 fruit, 30g	3	30	Low	1	Low

FOOD	SERVING SIZE	NET CARB (g)	GI VALUE	GI LEVEL	GL VALUE	GL LEVEL
Dragonfruit	½ fruit, 100g	6	30	Low	2	Low
Dried Apple	¼ cup, 28g	16	44	Low	10	Low
Dried Apricots Unsweetened	¼ cup, 32g	18	32	Low	12	med.
Dried Apricots Unsweetened	¼ cup, 32g	18	32	Low	12	med.
Dried Banana Unsweetened	¼ cup, 30g	22	54	Low	14	med.
Dried Banana Unsweetened	¼ cup, 30g	22	54	Low	14	med.
Dried Blueberries Unsweetened	¼ cup, 40g	26	53	Low	14	med.
Dried Cherries Unsweetened	¼ cup, 40g	30	54	Low	16	med.
Dried Coconut	¼ cup, 20g	7	40	Low	3	Low
Dried Cranberries Unsweetened	¼ cup, 40g	28	64	med.	18	med.
Dried Currants Unsweetened	¼ cup, 40g	30	56	med.	17	med.
Dried Custard Apple Unsweetened	¼ cup, 30g	22	48	Low	13	med.
Dried Custard Apple Unsweetened	¼ cup, 30g	22	48	Low	13	med.
Dried Dragon Fruit	¼ cup, 28g	15	57	med.	9	Low
Dried Goji Berries	¼ cup, 28g	14	29	Low	7	Low

FOOD	SERVING SIZE	NET CARB (g)	GI VALUE	GI LEVEL	GL VALUE	GL LEVEL
Dried Guava	¼ cup, 30g	18	45	Low	10	Low
Dried Kiwi Unsweetened	¼ cup, 30g	19	54	Low	11	med.
Dried Longan Unsweetened	¼ cup, 32g	28	54	Low	15	med.
Dried Lychee Unsweetened	¼ cup, 30g	22	52	Low	13	med.
Dried Mango Unsweetened	¼ cup, 30g	22	57	med.	12	med.
Dried Papaya Unsweetened	¼ cup, 30g	25	60	med.	15	med.
Dried Peach	¼ cup, 36g	20	35	Low	10	Low
Dried Pear Unsweetened	¼ cup, 40g	24	43	Low	12	med.
Dried Persimmon	¼ cup, 32g	24	53	Low	15	med.
Dried Pineapple Unsweetened	¼ cup, 35g	28	58	med.	16	med.
Dried Raspberries	¼ cup, 30g	16	40	Low	8	Low
Dried Sapodilla Unsweetened	¼ cup, 30g	20	50	Low	12	med.
Dried Strawberries	¼ cup, 30g	18	50	Low	10	Low
Fig Preserves	1 tbsp, 20g	13	54	Low	8	Low
Grape Jelly Homemade	1 tbsp, 20g	13	54	Low	8	Low
Grape Juice Concentrate	¼ cup, 60g	15	70	High	12	med.

FOOD	SERVING SIZE	NET CARB (g)	GI VALUE	GI LEVEL	GL VALUE	GL LEVEL
Grapefruit	1 med., 154g	13	30	Low	4	Low
Grapefruit Juice	½ cup, 120ml	11	48	Low	5	Low
Grapefruit segments Canned Light Syrup Drained	½ cup, 122g	10	25	Low	3	Low
Guava Canned Light Syrup Drained	½ cup, 122g	10	50	Low	5	Low
Guava Juice	½ cup, 120ml	10	33	Low	3.3	Low
Guava Nectar Canned Light	1 cup, 240g	30	45	Low	15	med.
Guava Sauce Cooked	1 cup, 250g	28	45	Low	14	med.
Lemon Curd Homemade	1 tbsp, 20g	13	54	Low	8	Low
Lemon Juice	½ cup, 120ml	10.5	20	Low	2	Low
Lemon Juice Concentrate	1 tbsp, 15g	1	20	Low	0.2	Low
Lime Juice Concentrate	1 tbsp, 15g	1	20	Low	0.2	Low
Mango Canned Light Syrup Drained	½ cup, 122g	16	50	Low	8	Low
Mango Jam	1 tbsp, 20g	13	54	Low	8	Low
Mango Juice	½ cup, 120ml	15	41	Low	6.2	Low
Mango Pickled	¼ cup, 60g	12	45	Low	6	Low

FOOD	SERVING SIZE	NET CARB (g)	GI VALUE	GI LEVEL	GL VALUE	GL LEVEL
Mixed Berry Jam	1 tbsp, 20g	13	54	Low	8	Low
Okra Pickled	1 cup, 160g	3	20	Low	1	Low
Orange Juice	½ cup, 120ml	13	50	Low	6.5	Low
Orange Marmalade Homemade	1 tbsp, 20g	13	54	Low	8	Low
Oranges Mandarin Canned Light Syrup Drained	½ cup, 122g	13	45	Low	6	Low
Papaya Canned Light Syrup Drained	½ cup, 122g	14	60	med.	7	Low
Passionfruit Juice	½ cup, 120ml	7	30	Low	2.1	Low
Passionfruit Juice Concentrate	¼ cup, 60g	8.7	35	Low	3	Low
Pawpaw	1 cup, 140g	11	60	med.	6	Low
Peach Juice	½ cup, 120ml	14	42	Low	6	Low
Peach Juice Concentrate	¼ cup, 60g	12	40	Low	6	Low
Peach Pickled	½ cup, 130g	16	45	Low	8	Low
Peach Preserves Homemade	1 tbsp, 20g	13	54	Low	8	Low
Peaches Canned Light Syrup Drained	½ cup, 122g	16	45	Low	8	Low
Pear Juice	½ cup, 120ml	14	44	Low	5.5	Low

FOOD	SERVING SIZE	NET CARB (g)	GI VALUE	GI LEVEL	GL VALUE	GL LEVEL
Pears Canned Extra Light Syrup	½ cup, 122g	11	45	Low	5.5	Low
Pears Canned Light Syrup Drained	½ cup, 122g	15	43	Low	7	Low
Peppers Pickled	1 cup, 150g	3	20	Low	1	Low
Pineapple Canned Extra Light Syrup	½ cup, 122g	15	54	Low	7.5	Low
Pineapple Frozen Chunks Sweetened	½ cup, 82g	21	58	med.	12.1	med.
Pineapple Juice	½ cup, 120ml	14	46	Low	6.5	Low
Pineapple Preserves	1 tbsp, 20g	14	55	Low	8	Low
Plum Jam	1 tbsp, 20g	13	54	Low	8	Low
Plum Pickled	1 cup, 150g	12	35	Low	6	Low
Plums Canned Extra Purple Light Syrup	½ cup, 122g	15	45	Low	6.7	Low
Plums Canned Light Syrup Drained	½ cup, 122g	12	40	Low	6	Low
Pomegranate Juice	½ cup, 120ml	17	53	Low	9	Low
Pomegranate Juice Concentrate	¼ cup, 60g	12	35	Low	8	Low
Prune Puree	¼ cup, 60g	24	45	Low	12	med.
Prune Whip	½ cup, 125g	28	45	Low	14	med.

FOOD	SERVING SIZE	NET CARB (g)	GI VALUE	GI LEVEL	GL VALUE	GL LEVEL
Purple Passion Fruit Juice	½ cup, 120ml	10	35	Low	5	Low
Quince Jelly	1 tbsp, 20g	13	54	Low	8	Low
Raspberries Canned Light Syrup Drained	½ cup, 122g	9	32	Low	3	Low
Raspberry Jam	1 tbsp, 20g	13	54	Low	8	Low
Raspberry Juice Concentrate	¼ cup, 60g	10	40	Low	5	Low
Red Currant Jelly	1 tbsp, 20g	13	54	Low	8	Low
Strawberry Jam	1 tbsp, 20g	13	54	Low	8	Low
Strawberry Juice Concentrate	¼ cup, 60g	10	40	Low	5	Low
Tomato Juice	1 cup, 240ml	10	38	Low	3.8	Low
Tsukemono Japanese Pickles	1 cup, 150g	4	20	Low	2	Low
Turnip Pickled	1 cup, 150g	3	20	Low	1	Low
Watermelon Juice	½ cup, 120ml	9	72	High	7.2	Low

10

GRAINS, CEREALS, PASTA & RICE

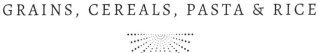

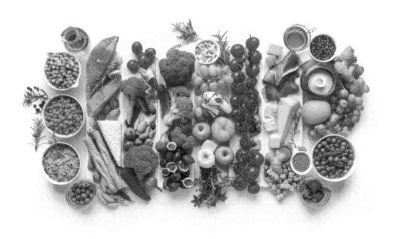

CARBOHYDRATE CONSIDERATIONS IN THE LOW-GL DIABETES DIET

Grains and cereals play a significant role in the Low-GL Diabetes Diet, and an analysis of their nutritional values is crucial for effective dietary management. Despite their integral role, most grains, cereals, and their products exhibit high Glycemic Load (GL) due to their high net carbohydrate content per standard serving size. The serving sizes listed are standard and not tailored to the guidelines of the Low-GL Diabetes Diet, which stipulate that one serving should contain no more than 15 grams of net carbohydrates.

To align with these guidelines, consider the following examples of grains with low glycemic Index (GI) values and calculate the portion sizes to fit the 15-gram net carb limit (see the following table for more details)

Whole Wheat Pasta:

- **GI Value**: Low (45)
- **Standard Serving Size**: 1 cup cooked (140g) yielding 49g net carbs.
- **Adjusted Serving Size**: Roughly ⅓ cup cooked to meet the 15g net carb requirement, minimizing the GL impact.

Egg Noodles:

- **GI Value**: Low (40)
- **Standard Serving Size**: 1 cup cooked (140g) yielding 50g net carbs.
- **Adjusted Serving Size**: About ⅓ cup cooked to fit the 15g net carb guideline, enhancing glycemic control.

These examples illustrate how reducing serving sizes can adapt high-carb foods to fit a low-GL dietary pattern, emphasizing that even small amounts of certain grains can contribute effectively to a diabetes-friendly diet without causing significant spikes in blood glucose.

FOOD	SERVING SIZE	NET CARB (g)	GI VALUE	GI LEVEL	GL VALUE	GL LEVEL
Amaranth	1 cup cooked (246g)	20g	35	Low	7	Low
Arrowroot Flour	1 cup (120g)	105g	69	Med.	33	High
Barley	1 cup cooked (157g)	32g	28	Low	9	Low
Barley Flour or Meal	1 cup (128g)	76g	55	Low	24	High
Barley Hulled	1 cup cooked (157g)	41g	30	Low	11	Med.
Barley Malt Flour	1 cup (122g)	84g	65	Med.	36	High
Bucatini	1 cup cooked (140g)	49g	45	Low	22	High
Buckwheat	1 cup cooked (168g)	33g	55	Low	15	Med.
Buckwheat	1 cup cooked (168g)	33g	55	Low	17	Med.
Buckwheat Flour Whole-Groat	1 cup (120g)	72g	50	Low	26	High
Buckwheat Groats	1 cup cooked (168g)	29g	45	Low	13	Med.
Buckwheat Porridge	1 cup cooked (168g)	23g	65	Med.	14	Med.
Bulgur	1 cup cooked (182g)	26g	46	Low	12	Med.
Congee	1 cup cooked (250g)	45g	76	High	30	High
Corn Bran Crude	1 cup (60g)	19g	45	Low	9	Low
Corn Flour Masa White	1 cup (114g)	77g	65	Med.	42	High

FOOD	SERVING SIZE	NET CARB (g)	GI VALUE	GI LEVEL	GL VALUE	GL LEVEL
Corn Flour Whole-Grain Blue	1 cup (128g)	76g	55	Low	34	High
Corn Flour Whole-Grain Yellow	1 cup (128g)	76g	55	Low	34	High
Corn Flour Degermed	1 cup (125g)	71g	55	Low	31	High
Corn Grain	1 cup cooked (164g)	45g	60	Med.	27	High
Cornmeal	1/4 cup dry (30g)	20g	69	Med.	15	Med.
Cornmeal Degermed	1 cup (138g)	75g	55	Low	32	High
Cornstarch	1 cup (128g)	107g	90	High	43	High
Couscous	1 cup cooked (157g)	36g	65	Med.	22	High
Cream of Wheat	1 cup cooked (244g)	26g	85	High	19	Med.
Eggplant Lasagna	1 cup (240g))	20g	50	Low	10	Low
Farina	1 cup cooked (242g)	26g	80	High	19	Med.
Farro	1 cup cooked (169g)	45g	40	Low	18	Med.
Four Cheese Lasagna	1 cup (240g))	20g	50	Low	8	Low
Freekeh	1 cup cooked (162g)	28g	43	Low	12	Med.
Garlic and Herb Penne	2 ounces (56g)	41g	50	Low	18	Med.
Gluten-Free Penne	2 ounces (56g)	43g	40	Low	10	Low
Grits	1 cup cooked (242g)	28g	80	High	15	Med.

FOOD	SERVING SIZE	NET CARB (g)	GI VALUE	GI LEVEL	GL VALUE	GL LEVEL
Hulled Barley	1 cup cooked (157g)	32g	28	Low	9	Low
Japanese Somen	1 cup (145g)	37g	50	Low	17	Med.
Kamut	1 cup cooked (172g)	45g	45	Low	20	High
Kamut Pasta	1 cup cooked (140g)	43g	50	Low	20	High
Mexican Lasagna	1 cup (240g))	35g	50	Low	15	Med.
Millet Flour	1 cup (120g)	87g	75	High	39	High
Millet Porridge	1 cup cooked (200g)	24g	70	High	14	Med.
Millet Raw	1 cup (200g)	82g	76	High	36	High
Multigrain Penne	2 ounces (56g)	41g	50	Low	11	Med.
Mushroom Lasagna	1 cup (240g))	33g	50	Low	13	Med.
Noodles, Brown Rice	1 cup cooked (180g)	40g	65	Med.	24	High
Noodles, Buckwheat	1 cup cooked (114g)	42g	45	Low	19	Med.
Noodles, Chow Mein	1 cup cooked (140g)	49g	45	Low	22	High
Noodles, Egg	1 cup cooked (140g)	50g	40	Low	20	High
Noodles, Gluten Free Corn	1 cup (200g)	42g	65	Med.	27	High
Noodles, Japanese Soba	1 cup cooked (140g)	44g	60	Med.	25	High
Noodles, Ramen	1 cup cooked (140g)	48g	46	Low	22	High

FOOD	SERVING SIZE	NET CARB (g)	GI VALUE	GI LEVEL	GL VALUE	GL LEVEL
Oat Bran	1 cup (94g)	44g	60	Med.	21	High
Oat Flour Partially Debranned	1 cup (120g)	69g	60	Med.	31	High
Oat Rolled	1 cup cooked (234g)	27g	57	Med.	15.4	Med.
Oats Steel-Cut	1 cup cooked (240g)	27g	54	Low	15	Med.
Pearled Barley	1 cup (157g)	41g	30	Low	11	Med.
Penne Ziti	2 ounces (56g)	41g	50	Low	18	Med.
Pesto Lasagna	1 cup (240g))	30g	50	Low	10	Low
Polenta	1 cup cooked (128g)	24g	85	High	18	Med.
Quinoa	1 cup cooked (185g)	34g	53	Low	10	Low
Quinoa Porridge	1 cup cooked (185g)	23g	65	Med.	13	Med.
Rice, Arborio	1 cup cooked (200g)	50g	70	High	33	High
Rice, Basmati	1 cup cooked (160g)	44g	65	Med.	24	High
Rice, Bhutanese Red	1 cup cooked (185g)	42g	55	Low	21	High
Rice, Black	1 cup cooked (186g)	45g	48	Low	16	Med.
Rice, Brown	1 cup cooked (195g)	42g	55	Low	22	High
Rice, Brown Basmati	1 cup cooked (195g)	45g	58	Med.	21	High

FOOD	SERVING SIZE	NET CARB (g)	GI VALUE	GI LEVEL	GL VALUE	GL LEVEL
Rice, Brown Jasmine	1 cup cooked (195g)	42g	60	Med.	22	High
Rice, Calrose	1 cup cooked (160g)	40g	75	High	28	High
Rice, Carnaroli	1 cup cooked (200g)	50g	70	High	33	High
Rice, Cream of	1 cup cooked (240g)	27g	85	High	20	High
Rice, Forbidden	1 cup cooked (186g)	45g	48	Low	16	Med.
Rice, Glutinous	1 cup cooked (174g)	42g	91	High	37	High
Rice, Jasmine	1 cup cooked (158g)	45g	74	High	29	High
Rice, Noodles	1 cup cooked (170g)	40g	55	Low	22	High
Rice, Red	1 cup cooked (185g)	42g	55	Low	21	High
Rice, Sushi	1 cup cooked (150g)	40g	80	High	30	High
Rice, Wehani	1 cup cooked (185g)	42g	55	Low	21	High
Rice, White	1 cup cooked (158g)	45g	78	High	29	High
Rice, Wild	1 cup cooked (164g)	32g	55	Low	16	Med.
Rye	1 slice of bread (32g)	14g	62	Med.	10	Low
Rye Flour Dark	1 cup (102g)	63g	45	Low	21	High
Rye Flour Light	1 cup (102g)	57g	45	Low	19	Med.

FOOD	SERVING SIZE	NET CARB (g)	GI VALUE	GI LEVEL	GL VALUE	GL LEVEL
Rye Flour Medium	1 cup (102g)	60g	45	Low	20	High
Rye Grain	1 cup cooked (174g)	31g	50	Low	14	Med.
Seafood Lasagna	1 cup (240g))	25g	50	Low	10	Low
Semolina	1 cup (167g)	97g	60	Med.	32	High
Semolina Porridge	1 cup cooked (167g)	22g	65	Med.	13	Med.
Soba	1 cup cooked (114g)	42g	45	Low	19	Med.
Sorghum	1 cup cooked (192g)	29g	65	Med.	19	Med.
Sorghum Flour Refined	1 cup (125g)	83g	70	High	33	High
Sorghum Grain	1 cup cooked (192g)	51g	69	Med.	30	High
Spaghetti Spinach Cooked	1 cup (140g)	49g	45	Med.	22	High
Spaghetti Spinach Dry	1 cup (100g)	70g	45	Low	31	High
Spaghetti, Buckwheat	1 cup cooked (140g)	42g	45	Low	19	Med.
Spaghetti, Capellini	1 cup cooked (140g)	49g	45	Low	22	High
Spaghetti, Carrot	1 cup cooked (140g)	49g	45	Low	22	High
Spaghetti, Gluten-Free	1 cup cooked (140g)	46g	52	Low	24	High
Spaghetti, Multigrain	1 cup cooked (140g)	46g	40	Low	18	Med.
Spaghetti, Spinach	1 cup cooked (140g)	49g	45	Low	22	High

FOOD	SERVING SIZE	NET CARB (g)	GI VALUE	GI LEVEL	GL VALUE	GL LEVEL
Spaghetti, Squid Ink	1 cup cooked (140g)	49g	45	Low	22	High
Spaghetti, Whole Wheat	1 cup cooked (140g)	45g	37	Low	17	Med.
Spaghetti, Zucchini (Zoodles)	1 cup (120g))	4g	15	Low	1	Low
Spelt	1 cup (194g)	44g	50	Low	24	High
Spelt Pasta	1 cup cooked (140g)	41g	49	Low	19	Med.
Spinach Lasagna	1 cup (240g))	30g	50	Low	12	Med.
Steel-Cut Oats	1 cup cooked (240g)	27g	55	Low	15	Med.
Sun-Dried Tomato Penne	2 ounces (56g)	41g	50	Low	18	Med.
Tapioca Pearl Dry	1 cup (152g)	122g	75	High	43	High
Teff	1 cup (252g)	42g	50	Low	17	Med.
Teff Porridge	1 cup cooked (240g)	29g	75	High	18	Med.
Traditional Lasagna	1 cup (240g))	36g	50		14	Med.
Tricolor Penne	2 ounces (56g)	41g	50		18	Med.
Triticale	1 cup cooked (182g)	40g	50	Low	19	Med.
Triticale Flour Whole-Grain	1 cup (120g)	72g	50	Low	27	High
Udon	1 cup cooked (160g)	52g	55	Low	28	High
Vegetarian Lasagna	1 cup (240g))	25g	50	Low	10	Low

FOOD	SERVING SIZE	NET CARB (g)	GI VALUE	GI LEVEL	GL VALUE	GL LEVEL
Vermicelli	1 cup cooked (140g)	49g	45	Low	22	High
Vermicelli Made From Soybeans	1 cup cooked (150g)	12g	25	Low	5	Low
Wheat Berries	1 cup cooked (198g)	45g	45	Low	20	High
Wheat Bran Crude	1 cup (58g)	20g	45	Low	7	Low
Wheat Durum	1 cup cooked (182g)	48g	50	Low	22	High
Wheat Flour Whole-Grain	1 cup (120g)	84g	65	Med.	36	High
Wheat Germ Crude	1 cup (115g)	39g	45	Low	15	Med.
Wheat Sprouted	1 cup (110g)	31g	50	Low	17	Med.
White Lasagna	1 cup (240g))	20g	50	Low	8	Low
Whole Grain Sorghum Flour	1 cup (125g)	83g	70	High	33	High
Whole Wheat Couscous	1 cup cooked (157g)	33g	55	Low	22	High
Whole Wheat Pasta	1 cup cooked (140g)	49g	45	Low	22	High
Whole Wheat Penne	2 ounces (56g)	39g	37	Low	7	Low

11

HERBS AND SPICES

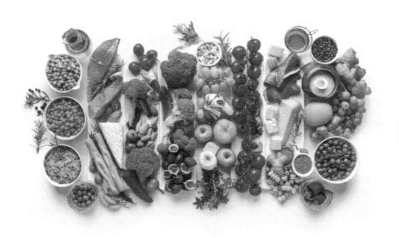

FOOD	SERVING SIZE	NET CARB (g)	GI VALUE	GI LEVEL	GL VALUE	GL LEVEL
Allspice	1 tsp, 2.1 g	1	15	Low	0.2	Low
Anise seeds	1 tsp, 2.1 g	1	0.0	Low	0	Low
Asian chives	1 tbsp, 3 g	1	15	Low	0.2	Low
Basil	1 tsp, 0.7 g	1	70	Low	0.7	Low
Bay leaves	1 tbsp, 1.8 g	0.6	23	Low	0.1	Low
Black cumin	1 tsp, 2.4 g	1	0.0	Low	0	Low
Black pepper	1 tsp, 2.4 g	1	44	Low	0.4	Low
capers	1 tbsp, 8.6 g	0.4	20	Low	0.1	Low
Caraway	1 tbsp, 6.7 g	1	5	Low	0.1	Low
Cardamom	1 tbsp, 5.8 g	1	82	Low	0.8	Low
Celery seed	1 tbsp, 5.8 g	1	32	Low	0.3	Low
Chiles	1 tbsp, 8 g	1	42	Low	0.4	Low
chili	1 tbsp, 8 g	1	15	Low	0.2	Low
Chives	1 tbsp, 2.8 g	1	15	Low	0.2	Low
Cinnamon	1 tbsp, 7.9 g	0.6	70	Low	0.4	Low
Cloves	1 tbsp, 6.6 g	1	87	Low	0.9	Low

FOOD	SERVING SIZE	NET CARB (g)	GI VALUE	GI LEVEL	GL VALUE	GL LEVEL
Coriander seed	1 tbsp, 5 g	1	33	Low	0.3	Low
Cumin	1 tbsp, 6 g	1.4	0.0	Low	0	Low
Curry Leaves	5 leaves, 2g	1	5	Low	0.1	Low
Curry powder	1 tbsp, 6 g	1	5	Low	0.1	Low
Dill seed	1 tsp, 2.4 g	1	15	Low	0.2	Low
Fennel seeds	1 tbsp, 5.8 g	0	16	Low	0	Low
Fenugreek	1 tbsp, 11.1 g	0.5	25	Low	0.1	Low
Fenugreek Leaves	1 cup, 85 g	3	25	Low	0.8	Low
Five Spice Powder	1 tsp, 2.1 g	1	15	Low	0.2	Low
Ginger	1 tsp, 2.1 g	1	72	Low	0.7	Low
Lemon Balm	1 tsp, 2.1 g	1	15	Low	0.2	Low
Lemongrass	1 cup, 67 g	5.5	45	Low	2.5	Low
Lime Leaves	5 leaves, 2 g	1	32	Low	0.3	Low
Mint	1 tbsp, 3.1 g	1	10	Low	0.1	Low
Mustard Seed	1 tsp, 2 g	1	32	Low	0.3	Low
Nutmeg	1 tsp, 2.4 g	1	46	Low	0.5	Low

FOOD	SERVING SIZE	NET CARB (g)	GI VALUE	GI LEVEL	GL VALUE	GL LEVEL
Oregano	1 tbsp, 3 g	1	5	Low	0.1	Low
Paprika	1 tsp, 2 g	0.5	15	Low	0.1	Low
Poppy seeds	1 tbsp, 8.8 g	0.4	5	Low	0	Low
Rosemary	1 tbsp, 3.3 g	1	70	Low	0.7	Low
Saffron	1 tsp, 0.7 g	1	70	Low	0.7	Low
Sage	1 tsp, 0.7 g	1	15	Low	0.2	Low
Savory	1 tbsp, 4.4 g	1	16	Low	0.2	Low
Sesame seeds	1 tbsp, 10 g	1	31	Low	0.3	Low
Sumac	1 tsp, 2.7 g	1	43	Low	0.4	Low
Tarragon	1 tbsp, 1.8g	1	15	Low	0.2	Low
Thyme	1 tbsp, 2.7 g	1	51	Low	0.5	Low
Turmeric	1 tbsp, 6.8 g	1.3	15	Low	0.2	Low
Vanilla	1 tbsp, 4.4 g	1	16	Low	0.2	Low
Wasabi powder	1 tsp, 2.8 g	2	31	Low	0.6	Low
Watercress	1 cup, 34 g	0.5	32	Low	0.2	Low
Wild garlic	1 oz, 28 g	3	11	Low	0.3	Low

12

NUTS & SEEDS

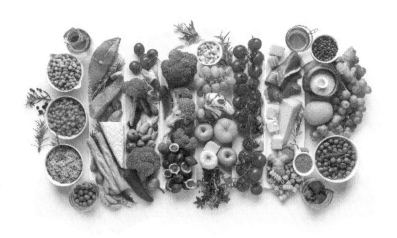

FOOD	SERVING SIZE	NET CARB (g)	GI VALUE	GI LEVEL	GL VALUE	GL LEVEL
Almond Butter	2 tbsp, 32g	3	10	Low	0.3	Low
Almonds Raw/Roasted	1 oz, 28g	2	7	Low	0.2	Low
Brazil Nut Butter	2 tbsp, 32g	2	15	Low	0.3	Low
Brazil nuts Raw/Roasted	1 oz, 28g	1	15	Low	0.2	Low
Butternuts	1 oz, 28g	2	15	Low	0.3	Low
Cashew Butter	2 tbsp, 32g	6	25	Low	1.5	Low
Cashews Raw/Roasted	1 oz, 28g	8	25	Low	2	Low
Chestnuts Boiled	1 oz, 28g	14	60	Med.	8.4	Low
Chestnuts Raw	1 oz, 28g	14	60	Med.	8.4	Low
Chestnuts Roasted	1 oz, 28g	14	60	Med.	8.4	Low
Chestnuts Steamed	1 oz, 28g	14	60	Med.	8.4	Low
Chia Nut Butter	2 tbsp, 32g	2	1	Low	0	Low
Chia Seeds Raw/Roasted	1 oz, 28g	2.2	5	Low	0.1	Low
Fennel seeds	1 oz, 28g	2	5	Low	0.1	Low
Fenugreek seeds	1 oz, 28g	6	15	Low	0.9	Low
Flaxseeds	1 oz, 28g	0	55	Low	0	Low
Hazelnut Butter	2 tbsp, 32g	3	15	Low	0.5	Low
Hazelnuts Raw/Roasted	1 oz, 28g	2	15	Low	0.3	Low

FOOD	SERVING SIZE	NET CARB (g)	GI VALUE	GI LEVEL	GL VALUE	GL LEVEL
Hemp seeds	1 oz, 28g	1	0	Low	0	Low
Macadamia Nut Butter	2 tbsp, 32g	3	15	Low	0.5	Low
Macadamia nuts Raw/Roasted	1 oz, 28g	2	15	Low	0.3	Low
Mustard seeds	1 oz, 28g	2	15	Low	0.3	Low
Peanut Butter	2 tbsp, 32g	6	20	Low	1.2	Low
Peanuts Raw/Roasted	1 oz, 28g	3	14	Low	0.4	Low
Pecans Raw/Roasted	1 oz, 28g	1	0	Low	0	Low
Pine nuts Raw/Roasted	1 oz, 28g	4	15	Low	0.6	Low
Pistachio Butter	2 tbsp, 32g	4	17	Low	0.6	Low
Pistachios Raw/Roasted	1 oz, 28g	5	15	Low	0.8	Low
Poppy seeds	1 oz, 28g	3	5	Low	0.2	Low
Pumpkin seeds	1 oz, 28g	2	15	Low	0.3	Low
Quinoa seeds	1 oz, 28g	4	53	Low	2.1	Low
Sesame seeds	1 oz, 28g	3	35	Low	1.1	Low
Sunflower seeds	1 oz, 28g	3	15	Low	0.5	Low
Tiger nuts	1 oz, 28g	11	51	Low	5.6	Low
Walnuts Raw/Roasted	1 oz, 28g	1	15	Low	0.2	Low
Watermelon seeds	1 oz, 28g	1	10	Low	0.1	Low

13

VEGETABLES & VEGETABLE PRODUCTS

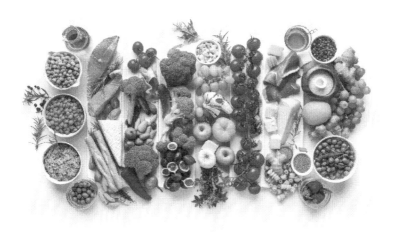

FOOD	SERVING SIZE	NET CARB (g)	GI VALUE	GI LEVEL	GL VALUE	GL LEVEL
Alfalfa Sprouts	1 cup, 33g	0.4	15	Low	1	Low
Amaranth Leaves	1 cup, 132g	5.4	65	Med.	4	Low
Artichoke	1 med., 120g	9	20	Low	3	Low
Artichoke {globe or french), raw	1 med., 120g	4.2	20	Low	4	Low
Arugula, raw	1 cup, 20g	0.4	30	Low	0	Low
Asparagus	1 cup, 134g	4	15	Low	1	Low
Avocado	½ fruit, 100g	2	15	Low	0	Low
Balsam-pear (bitter gourd), pods, raw	1 cup, 93g	2.3	25	Low	1	Low
Bamboo Shoots	1 cup, 151g	3	15	Low	1	Low
Bean Sprouts	1 cup, 104g	4	30	Low	2	Low
Beet Greens, Raw	1 cup, 144g	3	15	Low	1	Low
Beets, raw	1 cup, 136g	13	69	Med.	5	Low
Bell Peppers	1 cup, 149g	6	15	Low	1	Low
Bitter Melon	½ cup, 100g	4	30	Low	3	Low
Bok Choy, Raw	1 cup, 170g	1	15	Low	0	Low

FOOD	SERVING SIZE	NET CARB (g)	GI VALUE	GI LEVEL	GL VALUE	GL LEVEL
Borage, raw	1 cup, 89g	0.6	20	Low	1	Low
Broccoflower, Raw	1 cup, 100g	3	15	Low	1	Low
Broccoli	1 cup, 156g	6	15	Low	1	Low
Brussels Sprouts, Cooked	1 cup, 156g	8	15	Low	2	Low
Burdock root, raw	1 cup, 116g	14.3	50	Low	7	Low
Butternut Squash	1 cup, 205g	21	51	Low	8	Low
Cabbage Green, raw	1 cup, 205g	4	15	Low	1	Low
Cabbage, red, raw	1 cup, 89g	4	20	Low	1	Low
Cabbage, savoy, raw	1 cup, 70g	2.5	20	Low	1	Low
Cardoon, raw	1 cup, 120g	3.5	20	Low	1	Low
Carrot Greens	1 cup, 25g	1	15	Low	0	Low
Carrots, baby, raw	1 cup, 128g	11.5	54	Low	6	Low
Cassava	½ cup, 110g	39	46	Low	18	Med.
Cauliflower Greens	1 cup, 56g	2	15	Low	1	Low
Celeriac	1 cup, 156g	6	15	Low	1	Low
Celery	1 cup, 101g	2	15	Low	0	Low

FOOD	SERVING SIZE	NET CARB (g)	GI VALUE	GI LEVEL	GL VALUE	GL LEVEL
Chard, Raw	1 cup, 175g	5	15	Low	1	Low
Chayote, Raw	1 cup, 132g	4	15	Low	1	Low
Chicory greens, raw	1 cup, 55g	0.5	20	Low	1	Low
Chives	1 tbsp, 3g	0	15	Low	0	Low
Chrysanthemum leaves, raw	1 cup, 43g	0.6	20	Low	1	Low
Collard Greens	1 cup, 190g	5	15	Low	1	Low
Corn, sweet, white, raw	½ cup, 82g	19	60	Med.	11.4	Med.
Corn, sweet, yellow, raw	½ cup, 82g	19	60	Med.	11.4	Med.
Cress, garden, raw	1 cup, 25g	0.7	20	Low	1	Low
Cucumber, with peel, raw	1 cup, 104g	3	15	Low	1	Low
Daikon	1 cup, 116g	4	15	Low	1	Low
Dandelion Greens, Raw	1 cup, 55g	3	15	Low	1	Low
Dock, raw	1 cup, 133g	2	20	Low	1	Low
Drumstick pods, raw	1 cup, 99g	4	25	Low	2	Low
Edamame Unprepared	½ cup, 75g	8	15	Low	3	Low
Eggplant, Raw	1 cup, 99g	6	15	Low	1	Low
Endive Leaves	1 cup, 40g	1	15	Low	0	Low
Epazote, raw	1 cup, 20g	0.7	20	Low	1	Low

FOOD	SERVING SIZE	NET CARB (g)	GI VALUE	GI LEVEL	GL VALUE	GL LEVEL
Eppaw, raw	1 cup, 20g	1	20	Low	1	Low
Escarole	1 cup, 75g	3	15	Low	1	Low
Fennel Bulb	1 cup, 87g	5	15	Low	1	Low
Gourd, white-flowered (calabash), raw	1 cup, 116g	3	20	Low	1	Low
Grape leaves	1 cup, 28g	1.5	20	Low	1	Low
Green Onion	1 cup, 100g	4	15	Low	1	Low
Hearts of palm, raw	1 cup, 146g	4	20	Low	1	Low
Hubbard Squash	1 cup, 205g	16	50	Low	6	Low
Jalapeno	1 pepper, 14g	1	15	Low	0	Low
Jicama	1 cup, 120g	6	15	Low	2	Low
Jute, potherb, raw	1 cup, 28g	0.5	20	Low	1	Low
Kale	1 cup, 130g	4	15	Low	1	Low
Kelp	1 cup, 76g	1	15	Low	0	Low
Kohlrabi	1 cup, 135g	8	15	Low	2	Low
Lambsquarters, raw	1 cup, 28g	1	20	Low	1	Low
Leek Leaves	1 cup, 72g	4	15	Low	1	Low
Lemon grass (citronella), raw	1 tbsp, 6g	0.4	20	Low	1	Low

FOOD	SERVING SIZE	NET CARB (g)	GI VALUE	GI LEVEL	GL VALUE	GL LEVEL
Lettuce, green leaf, raw	1 cup, 36g	1	15	Low	1	Low
Lettuce, iceberg (includes crisphead types), raw	1 cup, 72g	1	15	Low	1	Low
Lettuce, red leaf, raw	1 cup, 28g	0.7	15	Low	1	Low
Lettuce, Romaine	1 cup, 72g	1	15	Low	1	Low
Lotus Root	1 cup, 120g	16	60	Med.	7	Low
Malabar spinach (Vine), raw	1 cup, 44g	0.8	20	Low	1	Low
Mushroom	1 cup, 70g	2	15	Low	0	Low
Nopales	1 cup, 86g	3	15	Low	1	Low
Okra	1 cup, 100g	4	15	Low	1	Low
Olives, Black	1 ounce, 28g	1	15	Low	0	Low
Olives, Green	1 ounce, 28g	1	15	Low	0	Low
Onions, spring or scallions, raw	1 cup, 100g	6	35	Low	3	Low
Onions, sweet, raw	1 cup, 160g	14	35	Low	5	Low
Onions, welsh, raw	1 cup, 100g	7	35	Low	3	Low
Parsley	1 tbsp, 3g	0	15	Low	0	Low
Parsnip	½ cup, 78g	12	52	Low	6	Low
Peppers, hot chili, green, raw	1 pepper, 14g	1	35	Low	1	Low

FOOD	SERVING SIZE	NET CARB (g)	GI VALUE	GI LEVEL	GL VALUE	GL LEVEL
Peppers, Hungarian, raw	1 cup, 125g	5	20	Low	1	Low
Peppers, jalapeno, raw	1 pepper, 14g	0.6	35	Low	1	Low
Peppers, serrano, raw	1 pepper, 18g	1	35	Low	1	Low
Peppers, sweet, green, raw	1 cup, 149g	6	20	Low	2	Low
Peppers, sweet, red, green, raw	1 cup, 149g	6	20	Low	2	Low
Potato, Cooked	½ cup, 105g	15	78	High	11	Low
Potatoes, flesh and skin, raw	1 med., 213g	33	65	Med.	18	Med.
Pumpkin leaves, raw	1 cup, 33g	0.6	20	Low	1	Low
Pumpkin, mashed	1 cup, 245g	9.3	78	High	7.5	Low
Purslane, raw	1 cup, 43g	0.7	20	Low	1	Low
Radish	1 cup, 116g	2	15	Low	0	Low
Rhubarb	1 cup, 122g	5	15	Low	1	Low
Rutabaga	½ cup, 85g	8	72	High	5	Low
Salsify, raw	1 cup, 133g	8	35	Low	3	Low
Seaweed, kelp, raw	1 cup, 36g	1	20	Low	1	Low
Seaweed, laver, raw	1 cup, 25g	1	20	Low	1	Low

FOOD	SERVING SIZE	NET CARB (g)	GI VALUE	GI LEVEL	GL VALUE	GL LEVEL
Seaweed, spirulina, raw	1 tbsp, 7g	0.3	20	Low	1	Low
Seaweed, wakame, raw	1 cup, 10g	0.5	20	Low	1	Low
Sesbania flower, raw	1 cup, 25g	1	20	Low	1	Low
Shallot	1 tbsp, 10g	2	15	Low	0.3	Low
Sorrel	1 cup, 29g	1	15	Low	0	Low
Spinach	1 cup, 180g	4	15	Low	0.6	Low
Squash Acorn	½ cup, 102g	15	75	High	7.5	Low
Squash Butternut	½ cup, 102g	21	51	Low	8	Low
Squash Spaghetti	1 cup, 155g	7	15	Low	1	Low
Sweet potato leaves, raw	1 cup, 28g	1	20	Low	1	Low
Sweet Potato, Boiled	1 serv., 75g	15	50	Low	7.5	Low
Sweet Potato, Roasted	1 serv., 75g	15	88	High	13.2	Low
Swiss Chard	1 cup, 175g	4	15	Low	1	Low
Taro leaves, raw	1 cup, 28g	1	20	Low	1	Low
Taro shoots, raw	1 cup, 84g	2	20	Low	1	Low
Taro, Tahitian, raw	½ cup, 104g	12.5	55	Low	9	Low
Tomatillo	1 cup, 132g	4	15	Low	1	Low

FOOD	SERVING SIZE	NET CARB (g)	GI VALUE	GI LEVEL	GL VALUE	GL LEVEL
Turnip	1 cup, 156g	8	62	Med.	4	Low
Waterchestnuts, chinese, raw	1 cup, 150g	24	60	Med.	9	Low
Watercress	1 cup, 34g	0	15	Low	0	Low
Yam, boiled	1 cup, 136 g	37	51	Low	18.9	Med.
Yam, fried	1 cup, 136 g	37	59	Med.	21.2	High
Yam, roasted	1 cup, 136 g	37	51	Low	18.9	Med.
Zucchini	1 cup, 124g	6	15	Low	2	Low

BIBLIOGRAPHY/REFERENCES

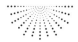

American Diabetes Association (2011). "Diagnosis and classification of diabetes mellitus." https://doi.org/10.2337/dc11-S062

Atkinson et al. (2014). "Type 1 diabetes." https://doi.org/10.1016/S0140-6736(13)60591-7

Beasley, Wylie-Rosett (2013)."The role of dietary proteins among people with diabetes." https://doi.org/10.1007/s11883-013-0348-2

Bjørgaas (2000). "Hypoglycemia--a dreaded complication of diabetes." https://pubmed.ncbi.nlm.nih.gov/11475234/

Blaak et al. (2021). "Carbohydrates: Separating fact from fiction." https://doi.org/10.1016/j.atherosclerosis.2021.03.025

Bornet et al. (1997). "Glycemic index concept and metabolic diseases." https://doi.org/10.1016/s0141-8130(97)00066-4

Campos et al. (2022) "Importance of Carbohydrate Quality: What Does It Mean and How to Measure It?" https://doi.org/10.1093/jn/nxac039

Chatterjee et al. (2017). "Type 2 diabetes." https://doi.org/10.1016/S0140-6736(17)30058-2

DeFronzo et al (2015). "Type 2 diabetes mellitus." https://doi.org/10.1038/nrdp.2015.19

Deshpande et al. (2008). "Epidemiology of diabetes and diabetes-related complications." https://doi.org/10.2522/ptj.20080020

DiMeglio et al., (2018). "Type 1 diabetes." https://doi.org/10.1016/S0140-6736(18)31320-5

Esposito et al. (2009) " Which diet is best for diabetes?" https://doi.org/10.1007/s00125-009-1292-0

Fletche (2002). "Risk factors for type 2 diabetes mellitus." https://doi.org/10.1097/00005082-200201000-00003

Flint et al. (2005)"The use of glycemic index tables to predict glycemic index of breakfast meals." https://doi.org/10.1079/bjn20041424

Forbes et al. (2013). "Mechanisms of Diabetic Complications." https://doi.org/10.1152/physrev.00045.2011

Frontoni et al. (2005). Papamichou et al. (2019)."Dietary patterns and management of type 2 diabetes" https://doi.org/10.1016/j.numecd.2019.02.004

Greenbaum (2002). "Insulin resistance in type 1 diabetes." https://doi.org/10.1002/dmrr.291

Großkopf, Simm (2024). "Carbohydrates in nutrition: friend or foe?" https://doi.org/10.1007/s00391-020-01726-1

Hamdy, Horton (2011)."Protein content in diabetes nutrition plan." https://doi.org/10.1007/s11892-010-0171-x

Harding et al. (2019). "Global trends in diabetes complications" https://doi.org/10.1007/s00125-018-4711-2

Jenkins et al. (1981). "Glycemic index of foods: a physiological basis for carbohydrate exchange." https://doi.org/10.1093/ajcn/34.3.362

Kalra et al. (2013). "Hypoglycemia: The neglected complication." https://doi.org/10.4103/2230-8210.117219

Khazrai et al. (2014) "Effect of diet on type 2 diabetes mellitus: a review." https://doi.org/10.1002/dmrr.2515

Kolarić et al. (2022). "Chronic Complications of Diabetes and Quality of Life." https://doi.org/10.20471/acc.2022.61.03.18

Malone (2019). "Does obesity cause type 2 diabetes mellitus (T2DM)? Or is it the opposite?." https://doi.org/10.1111/pedi.12787

Ndisang et al. (2017). "Insulin Resistance, Type 1 and Type 2 Diabetes, and Related Complications 2017." https://doi.org/10.1155/2017/1478294

Olsson et al. (2021). "Associations of carbohydrates and carbohydrate-rich foods with incidence of type 2 diabetes." https://doi.org/10.1017/S0007114520005140

Papamichou et al. (2019)."Dietary patterns and management of type 2 diabetes" https://doi.org/10.1016/j.numecd.2019.02.004

Petersmann et al. (2019). "Definition, Classification and Diagnosis of Diabetes Mellitus." https://doi.org/10.1055/a-1018-9078

Rivellese et al. (2012). "Dietary carbohydrates for diabetics." https://doi.org/10.1007/s11883-012-0278-4

Sawyer, Gale (2009). "Diet, delusion and diabetes." https://doi.org/10.1007/s00125-008-1203-9

Seckold et al. (2018)"The ups and downs of low-carbohydrate diets in the management of Type 1 diabetes" https://doi.org/10.1111/dme.13845

Shkembi et al., 2023. Glycemic Responses of Milk and Plant." https://www.ncbi.nlm.nih.gov/pmc/articles/PMC9914410/

Slavin JL, Lloyd B. (2012). "Health Benefits of fruits and vegetables." https://doi.org/10.3945/an

Slavin, Carlson (2014). "Carbohydrates" https://doi.org/10.3945/an.114.006163

Solis-Herrera et al. (2021). "Pathogenesis of Type 2 Diabetes Mellitus." https://www.ncbi.nlm.nih.gov/books/NBK279115/

Taylor (2013). "Type 2 diabetes: etiology and reversibility." https://doi.org/10.2337/dc12-1805.

Vasiljevic et al. (2020). "The making of insulin in health and disease." https://doi.org/10.1007/s00125-020-05192-7

Vinik, Jenkins (1988) "Dietary fiber in management of diabetes." https://doi.org/10.2337/diacare.11.2.160

Widanagamage et al. (2009). "Carbohydrate-rich foods: glycemic index and the effect of constituent macronutrients." https://doi.org/10.1080/09637480902849195.

Wilcox (2005). "Insulin and insulin resistance." https://www.ncbi.nlm.nih.gov/pmc/articles/PMC1204764/

Wolever et al. (1992). "Beneficial effect of a low glycemic index diet in type 2 diabetes." https://doi.org/10.1111/j.1464-5491.1992.tb01816.x

Workeneh, Mitch (2013)."High-protein diet in diabetic nephropathy: what is really safe?" https://doi.org/10.3945/ajcn.113.067223

Yen, et al. (2022). "Increased vegetable intake improves glycemic control in adults with type 2 diabetes mellitus." https://doi.org/10.2337/dc11-S062

Zhou et al. (2022). "Gut Microbiota: An Important Player in Type 2 Diabetes Mellitus." https://doi.org/10.3389/fcimb.2022.834485

HEALTH AND NUTRITION WEBSITES

- Centers for Disease Control and Prevention: https://www.cdc.gov/healthyweight
- Fruits and Vegetables Matter: https://www.fruitsandveggiesmatter.gov
- Cooking Light: https://www.cookinglight.com
- Nutrition.gov: https://www.nutrition.gov
- Hormone Foundation: https://www.hormone.org
- American Diabetes Association: https://www.diabetes.org
- American Heart Association: https://www.americanheart.org
- National Institute on Aging: https://www.nia.nih.gov
- National Institutes of Health: http://health.nih.gov
- National Kidney Disease Education Program | NIDDK: https://www.niddk.nih.gov/health-information/community-health-outreach/information-clearinghouses/nkdep
- American Kidney Fund (AKF): https://www.kidneyfund.org/
- The National Institute of Diabetes and Digestive and Kidney Diseases (NIDDK): https://www.niddk.nih.gov/health-information/kidney-disease

ABOUT THE AUTHOR

Dr. H. Maher" is a joint pen name under which Dr. Y. Naitlho, PharmD (Doctor of Pharmacy), and H. Naitlho, MEng (ISAE-SUPAERO), MEng (École de l'Air et de l'Espace), Advanced MSc (Paul Sabatier University), and Executive MBA, co-write books.

Dr. Y. Naitlho, PharmD, brings over 25 years of experience in pharmacy practice, with a special emphasis on nutrition, healthy eating, and writing. He obtained his Doctor of Pharmacy degree from the Perm State Pharmaceutical Academy in 1998. Dr. Y. Naitlho is notably active within the healthcare community, particularly through his community pharmacy. He, along with his pharmacy team, spearheads patient education initiatives, providing medication counseling, printed educational materials, and advice on dietary regulation, exercise, and lifestyle adjustments for patients managing chronic diseases such as diabetes, hypertension, heart disease, and kidney disorders.

Additionally, Dr. Y. Naitlho participates in humanitarian campaigns in collaboration with multidisciplinary healthcare professionals, including endocrinologists, cardiologists, ophthalmologists, and nephrologists. This joint effort is designed to deliver comprehensive support to those in need, ensuring they receive the most effective and optimal care available.

H. Naitlho possesses over 30 years of experience in engineering, operations, project management, as well as in scientific and engineering research. He is an established author of several books on business management and a co-author of a vast array of publications on food science, human nutrition, food engineering, and applied nutrition. H. Naitlho earned a Master of Systems Engineering from the École Nationale Supérieure d'Aéronautique et de l'Espace (ISAE-SUPAERO), a Master in Aeronautical Systems Engineering from the French Air and Space Force Academy, an Advanced Master in Automatics from Paul Sabatier University, and an additional Master's degree in Mechanical Engineering from Aix Marseille University, alongside an Executive MBA from Laureate International Universities. His engineering mindset and scientific rigor enhance their collaborative work, demonstrating a meticulous approach to refining ideas, analyzing data, and ensuring consistency and attention to detail in their writing projects.

Together, Dr. Y. Naitlho and H. Naitlho share a profound commitment to assisting individuals with diabetes, chronic kidney disease (CKD), and hypertension in leading healthier, more satisfying lives through informed food choices and customized meal plans. They are dedicated to keeping abreast of the latest research and nutritional guidelines to furnish their readers with accurate, dependable, and actionable information. Their combined efforts culminate in books that empower those with these health conditions to take control of their health and savor a diverse, nutritious diet.

70419117R00149